MELT
PERFORMANCE

Also by Sue Hitzmann

The MELT Method: A Breakthrough Self-Treatment System to Eliminate Chronic Pain, Erase the Signs of Aging, and Feel Fantastic in Just 10 Minutes a Day!

Sue Hitzmann

MELT

PERFORMANCE

A Step-by-Step Program to
Accelerate Your Fitness Goals,
Improve Balance and Control,
and Prevent Chronic Pain and
Injuries for Life

 HarperOne
An Imprint of HarperCollins Publishers

HarperOne

HarperCollins books may be purchased for educational, business, or sales promotional use. For information, please email the Special Markets Department at SPsales@harpercollins.com.

FIRST EDITION

Photographs by Brian Leighton
Illustrations by Gene Clark

Library of Congress Cataloging-in-Publication Data

Names: Hitzmann, Sue, author.
Title: Melt performance : a step-by-step program to accelerate your fitness goals, improve balance and control, and prevent chronic pain and injuries for life / Sue Hitzmann.
Description: First edition. | New York, NY : HarperOne, [2019] | Includes bibliographical references and index.
Identifiers: LCCN 2019004756 | ISBN 9780062882424 (hardback)
Subjects: LCSH: Chronic pain—Treatment—Popular works. | Self-care, Health—Popular works. | BISAC: HEALTH & FITNESS / Pain Management. | HEALTH & FITNESS / Healing. | MEDICAL / Allied Health Services / Massage Therapy.
Classification: LCC RB127 .H582 2019 | DDC 616/.0472—dc23 LC record available at https://lccn.loc.gov/2019004756

19 20 21 22 23   LSC   10 9 8 7 6 5 4 3 2 1

For Leon Chaitow,

for teaching me the importance

of thinking outside the box

Contents

PART THREE
NeuroStrength Performance Sequences

PART FOUR
NeuroStrength Performance Maps

Contents

Foreword

I was honored when Sue Hitzmann asked me to write the foreword to *MELT Performance*. I respect Sue's prolific work as a writer, thinker, and exercise physiologist who continues to modernize the fitness industry with her innovative blend of connective tissue and nervous system techniques. The nervous system has the rare ability to record our responses to life events. With repetition, these responses become fixed in living tissue. When an event such as an injury occurs, the recorded response may be vital in the moment but not suited for long-term success. Like an orchestra, each part of the body is related, and when one section goes off-key, the rest of the group jumps in to compensate. The goal of this supportive compensation is to attain the most balance possible for maximum operational support in the moment. However, problems arise when we continue to use neurological compensations long after an injury has healed. This is where Sue's NeuroStrength self-care program can help. By recognizing the connection, function, and structure of connective tissue in the body, NeuroStrength allows us to assess and treat altered brain maps that may be causing compensations and, in turn, leading to loss of spinal and pelvic stability and efficient motor control. Thickening, snagging, or holding in any part of the connective-tissue web results in a general heaviness of movement. What begins as a way to protect the body (particularly a part that hurts) eventually results in reduced fluidity throughout the entire body. One of the hardest things to do in a presentation or in print is to take complex topics and make them simple. This book does just that. *MELT Performance* is written in a way that educates the novice *and* the experienced trainer. Sue provides a user-friendly road map that teaches us to evaluate our strengths and weaknesses more objectively—and take the necessary action to make lasting changes.

What strikes me most about Sue's work is the method and quality of thinking. As you explore her blogs, articles, interviews, bestselling book *The MELT Method*, and this newest book, it becomes apparent that all these pieces come together to form a cohesive whole. Everything from pain reduction, biomechanics, and the sensorimotor system to psychology, strength training, and athletic movement is eloquently blended. Thus, *MELT Performance* provides one-stop shopping for a total-body training program. The work itself has the bracing clarity that comes from thinkers who spend their entire lives in direct empirical engagement with a subject they love. Sue approaches her subject with as much humility and as few preconceived notions as possible. Her ideas emerge from observation and not vice versa. What works for Sue and her students comes to the fore. Everything else drops away. What remains is a humane, flexible, systematic, and nondogmatic approach. The job becomes, as often attributed to Albert Einstein, "as simple as possible, but no simpler."

Whenever I find such thinkers, I cling to their work—not just for what I can learn about the subject at hand but for what I can learn about how to live, how to think, and how to approach life. If you're like me, as you read through these chapters, you'll feel a growing compulsion to make your body better and to make *you* better.

It's been said you should seek out and study people who have "been there and done that." I believe it's better to study with those who have been there, done that, and are *still* doing it! No one in the fitness business has Sue's breadth of quality and experience. She has tried everything, improved everything, and come to more fitness "eureka" moments than anyone around. In an industry that changes so fast, you need to keep up with people who *stay* on the cutting edge—people like Sue Hitzmann.

In *MELT Performance*, Sue teaches us how to get ahead of the factors that contribute to injury and pain so we can perform at our highest level. She makes clear that optimum health requires a seamless continuum of proactive care, not just reactive rehab. I hope this work changes your perspective on health care. You should have the mindset that you, both personally and professionally, are a powerful player in the quest to get upstream of lifestyle-induced stress and injury conditions. By following Sue's protocols, we can upgrade our lives and accelerate quality outcomes for all.

—Erik Dalton, PhD,
founder of the Freedom From Pain Institute
and author of *Dynamic Body: Exploring
Form, Expanding Function*

MELT
PERFORMANCE

Introduction

Beyond Fitness

Are you dedicated to living a healthy, active lifestyle but constantly dealing with joint aches, tendon or ligament strains, or muscle pains that make it harder and harder to reach your fitness goals?

Are you an athlete striving to be at the top of your game but facing repeated injuries that hold you back?

Are you ready to be active and exercise regularly without worrying about injuries or muscle and joint damage?

Then you are ready for MELT Performance, a revolutionary new method that applies the most cutting-edge science and research to maximize and accelerate your fitness goals. For anyone looking to achieve peak performance, this technique will help you reach your goals faster, improve balance and control, and reduce your risk of injuries and your chances of having persistent pain—for good.

MELT Performance is the missing link that will transform your body from the inside out. I'm going to teach you about a very vital but overlooked key to unlocking your ability to sustain your athleticism and maximize your results. The secret is neurological stability—or what I call NeuroStrength.

Stability seems like something that regular sports and exercise training would improve. Yet one of the most common roadblocks to leading an active lifestyle is sustaining a stress injury or managing chronic joint pain or muscle strains. When I see clients who have hurt themselves being active, they often say, "I wasn't even doing anything out of the ordinary!" Why is it that you can practice the same pitch, the same swing, the same Downward Dog, or the same pirouette for years, yet somehow, suddenly, for no reason, that movement causes a sudden pain in your back or your knee? When you've done these movements skillfully, thousands of times already, why did that last one cause pain?

There is a little-known problem that affects anyone dedicating time and effort to staying in shape, playing sports, or performing at the peak of their ability. Whether or not you're an athlete in training, if you're dedicated to leading an active lifestyle—through running, cycling, practicing your backhand, doing training drills, or even perfecting a yoga pose—you practice and repeat movements over and over to improve your performance. And if you're like me, when you meet your goals, you train harder and set even higher goals.

The problem is that the repetition required to continuously improve how you move has a downside. Whether you're an Olympic athlete or a weekend warrior, 80 percent of orthopedic injuries happen because of repetitive stress, *not* accidents. Even professional athletes who have a net worth of hundreds of millions of dollars from endorsements—and who have access to the best therapists, technology, and supplements—still sustain injuries all the time. Constant training for a sport creates patterns. Think of patterns like your favorite pair of jeans. After you wear them a hundred times, they deform and lose their perfect fit as the denim loses its elastic recoil. Repetition causes connective tissue to endure repeated tension and compression in local regions that, over time, can cause global instabilities—and that causes your body to compensate.

So although more exercise means fewer obesity-related diseases, exercise-related injuries may negate the upside of engaging in an active lifestyle. In any given year, more than half of people who work out to keep themselves fit have a stress injury—a strained muscle, a sprained ligament, or a torn tendon causing joint damage. And here's a secret: Athletes are more likely to be injured while *training*—not while competing in their sport!

Why does this happen? Why is that 80 percent figure so high? Because the current model of *how* to exercise—whether for amateurs or for seasoned professionals—hasn't yet caught up to the cutting-edge theories of MELT Performance. That's not to say that coaches, trainers, and physical therapists don't know what they're doing. Usually, they do. It's just that MELT Performance is a new way to move. To retrain your brain. And to create the kind of neurological stability in your body that will prevent these injuries from happening.

In addition, psychological factors, especially stress, are important antecedents to injuries. Stress and psychology play significant roles in injury rehab and can make or break successful return-to-play for many athletes and casual exercisers. I see this when I watch professional athletes in motion and can instantly tell from how they serve at tennis or how they swing a baseball bat whether their pelvis or shoulder girdle is out of balance or lacks stability. They're strong and tough and expert, but they just do not have the kind of stability that MELT Performance can give them. After my decades of experience with hands-on bodywork, I can both see these imbalances and am able to predict what kind of injury the athlete will be prone to should he or she continue without restoring neurological stability. The problem is, movement repetition is so common that few people consider that the reason they sprained an ankle was because their hips were unstable—not just because of sports-specific training but because of the mixture of repetitive postures and movements of their daily lives.

No matter how strong you become or how hard you train, repetition is the blessing and the curse of all athletic performance. Your body gets used to what you do and how you move, and it creates compensatory patterns to reserve energy and effort— until it can't anymore. That's when you stand up and wonder why your back is so sore, or why you don't have any energy at the end of the day, or why you keep getting hurt when you're working out.

It's not just that repetition increases your risk of injury; it actually gets in the way of achieving peak performance. No matter what your level of exercise experience, I am not asking you to stop training or working out; instead, I want to share with you my incredibly simple method to address the effects of repetition and give you a competitive, lifelong advantage.

We've been told countless times that what keeps us stable and upright is the strength of our muscles and the alignment of our bones. So if we exercise to keep our muscles strong, eat right, and do things that improve our bone density, we will stay fit, healthy, and energetically balanced, right? Wrong!

As a society, we've bought in to the belief that the key to peak performance is muscle strength. However, as we train, repetition can both improve functional motor skills *and* cause abnormal movement patterns caused by accumulated stress. These abnormal movements cause restrictions that lead to compensatory patterns. The term *common compensatory pattern* was coined by Dr. J. Gordon Zink to describe commonly found patterns of dysfunction in the body. The concept of neuromyofascial-skeletal units and measuring recurring patterns of dysfunction have been aspects of my clinical research for decades. What I can tell you is, no matter how strong you are, *repetition causes compensatory patterns* that can lead to instability in your joints and interfere with your overall muscle timing—and you don't even know that this compensation is happening. Instead, we wait until an injury occurs, and even then, many physical therapists will focus on the injury rather than on the instability that caused it. I'm going to show you what this instability looks and feels like in your own body, even help you identify compensatory patterning existing in your own body, and together we are going to reverse it.

The fact is, whether you're a pro athlete, someone who goes to the gym regularly, or someone who just walks the dog several times a day, exercise and strength training don't necessarily improve stability. It just doesn't work that way. When you are fit and engaging in a healthy lifestyle, you might think your body is stable, but over time, the stability and alignment of your joints can be compromised by the repetitive movements you're always doing.

When we have instability, we don't *not* move; we just don't move as accurately as is considered "ideal." For example, you work at your desk staring at a computer screen all day. You use a mouse with your right hand, and you frequently cross your right leg over your left leg, and your left foot is often on part of the chair rather than on the floor. This causes your right hip to be under more tension laterally, and the left foot and thigh are more weighted and compressed. When you stand up, your pelvis is still torqued, like it was when you were sitting. This causes adaptations in your lower back and pelvic stability. You walk anyway, you move anyway, but your back always hurts.

Compensation is inefficient—and exhausting. Often, when athletes feel exhausted, they actually push themselves to train harder, because they've been told that pushing harder makes them stronger. But then they only get more tired. The more you deplete your body, the more you make yourself exhausted and prone to injuries because your foundation is unstable and you haven't known how to fix it. We fail to realize that as stress accumulates, our bodies never give up—they compensate so we can keep going.

There is a vital system that supports, protects, and stabilizes the entire body—the *connective tissue* or *fascial system.* Every organ, muscle, tendon, ligament, nerve, cell, and molecule in your body functions within this three-dimensional, body-wide stability system. Fascia is everywhere—a seamless, three-dimensional system; a mesh-like, microscopic tissue comprised of cells, gels, and fibers that connects everything and gives our form its shape. Under a microscope, fascia's collagen fibrils (liquid-lined, hollow fibers) look like a liquid spider's web. However, everything from repetitive daily postures and movements to injury and disease can cause this tissue to appear more like a cobweb, tacked down and less able to allow for the necessary gliding at the interfaces of all structures such as nerves, muscles, and tendons. Recent research is proposing that collagen acts like a superconductor. The continuum of fascia throughout the body allows it to serve as a body-wide mechanosensitive signaling system, and it plays an important role in proprioception. Information from the body is sent to the brain in two ways: by sensory fibers at speeds from 2 to 100 meters per second or as mechanical vibrations within the fascia at the speed of sound—1,500 meters per second, far faster than nerve impulses travel. Technology is allowing us to measure the bioelectrical pathophysiological regulation of the connective tissue matrix. Stimulating tissue in one area of the matrix, like a spider's web, will cause an effect through the entire web, for better and sometimes for worse. Without fascia being able to slide and glide, inflammation and irritation are inevitable during movement and cell to cell communication declines. Connective tissue is designed to stabilize joints and provide muscle support, connection, and integration so we move efficiently. But our repetitive movements and postures cause excessive tension and compression on this tissue, which causes it to lose its supportive, flexible properties. The more we repeat a motion or posture, the more the integrity of this tissue is challenged. This is a key contributor to muscle weakness, aches and pains, and a decline in performance, which can lead to an array of physical dysfunction and emotional issues.

In other words, whether you're practicing a golf swing for hours or sitting at a desk all day, *repetition slowly causes connective tissue to adapt*, and when it does, it loses its fluid flow, or hydration, on a cellular level. Hydration is essential for connective tissue to provide supple stability. I call this cellular deformation *stuck stress.* Much like sediment in a river, this dehydration and deformation accumulates. And when it does, it causes a dysfunctional cascade that can't be addressed by diet and exercise alone.

The big issue for performance is that *stuck stress affects your neurological stability and control systems.* When stability declines, compensation begins. That's why so many people who exercise and eat right still have joint pain, chronic body issues, and are energetically fatigued—even those who are in shape. We blame aging for these issues, but they're actually caused by accumulated stuck stress. Stability is the key for staying injury-free and for reaching peak performance.

As a clinician I frequently find recurrent patterns caused by fascial bias—an overlooked element of instability, imbalance, postural misalignments, and motor timing. Andrew Taylor Still, the founder of osteopathy, once said, "Fascia is the place to look for the cause of disease and the place to consult and begin the action of remedies in all diseases." Every bone, muscle, nerve, and organ develops within and is covered with fascia, thus fascia's inherent link to movement is obvious once you understand that it is the most abundant, supportive material in the body.

For example, a baseball pitcher always posts on the same leg, rotates in one direction, and throws a pitch with the same arm. This repetition causes fascia to adapt, and the pitcher gets really good at throwing a ball. But this fascial adaptability can also lead to some muscles getting tight and overpowering, while others get elongated and inhibited. A common injury among pitchers is damage to a forearm ligament (the ulnar collateral ligament), often leading to what's called Tommy John surgery. Pitchers don't realize that while they are getting good at throwing a ball accurately, their upper and lower body instabilities and fascial adaptability leave them and their elbow susceptible to excessive torque, ultimately leading to this horrible injury. You don't just tear a thick ligament out of nowhere. The accumulative, repeated pitching strains the supportive potential and elastic properties of the tissues until they just can't do their job well. Then the pitcher becomes injured and may never pitch again—and certainly never as well as before surgery. The psychological damage this causes can often lead to other issues, too.

In my first book, *The MELT Method*, I introduced techniques that focus on rehydrating your connective tissues and rebalancing the nervous system to eliminate stuck stress and improve whole-body efficiency. That book helped hundreds of thousands of people break free from chronic pain. The basic methods covered in *The MELT Method* are the launchpad for what we will be doing in *MELT Performance*. *MELT Performance* takes this a step farther to help you reacquire neurological stability, improve your foundation, and achieve pain-free, high-level performance in all your physical activities, with no downside.

The good news is that restoring stability is easy if you know how to do it. This book contains everything you need to know to gain the competitive advantage you have been looking for. It's also an insurance policy for anyone who wants to enjoy a pain-free, active lifestyle.

MELT Performance will improve your neurological stability so you can train smarter, not harder. Although the moves might look easy, you're going to be shocked by how little control and stability you actually have and how much you compensate without even being aware of it.

You will learn why neurological stability is so vital to your performance. Without it, you simply reinforce your existing instability and strengthen your compensatory patterns during your workouts—becoming a stronger but a more unstable body. You basically get better at managing instability until pain or injury slows you down and you lose all of your short-term gains.

MELT Performance will help you break this cycle. Not only will you eliminate unnecessary muscle compensation and save your joints, but you will unleash your body's peak performance for optimal results, allowing you to reach even bigger goals. This will give you the secret to lifelong activity, allowing you to continue to do the things you love to do, whenever you want to do them.

MELT Performance is not exercise. It doesn't replace anything in your current routine; it enhances everything else you already do. It directly addresses aspects of your body that no training regimen, diet, or medicine can affect. It's a game-changer and a life-changer.

Even better, MELT Performance is a maintenance program that takes only a few minutes a day. I've even created training- and game-day MELT Maps to take the guesswork out of which moves, in which order, will best serve your specific needs (see Chapter 11). On game days you obviously have limited time, so you'll take only ten to fifteen minutes either in the morning or up to one hour before game time rehydrating your fascia and giving it a little boost in its supportive qualities. Training Day MELT Maps enhance your shoulder and hip stability and establish efficient core control. These Maps should precede your sports-specific training routines, and they can also help prevent common injuries in your sport if you use them on your recovery days. They take fifteen to thirty minutes of your training time—but you only need to do them a minimum of *once* every week to feel results.

I've also devised the basic protocols for specific joint injuries and the best MELT Maps to restore function and eliminate pain. These are great recovery Maps to do at the end of a day so you wake up the next morning with less accumulated stress in your joints and start your day off on the right foot. Finally, because the repetitive postures and movements of daily living exist even when we aren't playing a sport, I've created Lifestyle Maps for after a long day spent sitting on buses or planes traveling from event to event.

Whether you're a world-class sports star or a weekend warrior, MELT Performance has an even more powerful element. When I say "athlete," I really mean your inner spirit or your inner warrior. A person who trains regularly for or is skilled in a sport or game requiring physical strength, agility, or stamina can certainly be called an athlete. But even an athlete has a life beyond his or her sport.

Having worked in the fitness business for nearly thirty years, I've learned how an athlete's mindset is often more important than his or her natural athletic talent. When you are an athlete, you not only condition your body for the sport, but you condition your mind as well. Molding young athletes with positive characteristics and life skills that will serve them beyond their athletics is often missing in basic sports coaching and training. Whether you are a professional athlete or someone who just wants to be fit and athletic, I want to help you add those all-important emotional skills back into your routine and life. Had I known as a teen athlete what I know now, I'd have been able to push myself to my full potential without the risk of being injured yet again.

MELT Performance will help improve your balance, control, and agility; prevent chronic pain and injuries; wake up your brain; improve your circulation, sleep, longevity, and overall resilience; and undo years of emotional holding and habits that may have held you back from your true potential.

If you want to live a long, healthy, active, pain-free life, then MELT Performance is for you. It is going to transform your body and your results for years to come.

▶ The Prequel of MELT, or How MELT Performance Came to Be

I admit it. I am a total science geek, and I love sharing science with other people. But human biology and physiology are complex. My goal is to help my clients solve their chronic pain and improve their performance, and I've spent decades simplifying the inner workings of the human body so they can understand how MELT works.

MELT Performance is so different from anything you've ever tried—and the results are so profound—that I'm sure you're curious about *how* it works. The good news is that you don't have to know the specifics to reap the benefits. If you want to jump into the moves and sequences in Part Two and Part Three of this book, and experience my geek-out science explanations in Part One later, feel free!

In *The MELT Method*, I explained the missing link to pain-free living—healthy, hydrated connective tissue and a balanced nervous system. I also gave you the protocol to rehydrate your connective tissue and restore whole-body balance, which I call the Four Rs of MELT—Reconnect, Rebalance, Rehydrate, and Release. This is the ideal protocol for eliminating stuck stress and getting the regulators of your nervous system back on track, which is the secret to getting out of chronic pain. You can read all about the Four Rs in Chapter 4, because these techniques are the foundation of the MELT Performance sequences.

In fact, I developed the process of what I call Hands-Off Bodywork in reverse order. The Two Rs of NeuroStrength—Reintegrate and Repattern—did in fact precede the development and creation of the MELT Method. Long before I created MELT, I was looking for ways to simulate the brilliant hands-on neuromuscular therapy techniques that I learned from the naturopath, osteopath, and manual therapist Leon Chaitow. Neuromuscular therapy is a highly specialized type of hands-on soft-tissue therapy designed to relieve pain and return injured tissues to normal function. It utilizes specific, targeted soft-tissue treatments to eliminate the causes of most muscular aches and pains. This form of hands-on therapy requires a therapist to be able to palpate tissue for stiffness, mobility, and sensitivity. Muscle testing is used to determine which muscles are perhaps faulty in their activation or release. The body is treated first by assessing tissue tone, then manually turning on inhibited stabilizers, and regaining their recruitment and activation while also releasing unnecessary contraction or overly engaged muscle movers. Tissue tone is then reassessed for improved joint motion.

In twenty-plus years of practicing these techniques, I was able to provide pain relief for people where more traditional stretching and strength approaches had failed. I realized that there was far more to overall function and efficiency than basic exercise techniques. Neuromuscular therapy balances the nervous system with the muscular and skeletal systems and naturally brings the body back into alignment. It addresses postural and muscular imbalances, nerve entrapment, ischemia (reduced blood flow to an area of the body), and what are often called muscular trigger points.

Although neuromuscular therapy is the most effective way I have ever seen to restore function after a sports injury or acute trauma without surgery or medicine, most coaches, trainers, and doctors aren't familiar with it. If it's used at all, it's during rehab, not *pre*-hab—that is, *before* someone is injured or feeling a decline in their athletic resilience. Athletes in training regularly work with coaches, but they use a physical therapist only if they are having a problem. Why do we wait for injuries to occur before we intervene in repetitive stress? For all the money team owners spend on marketing and business expenses, you'd think they'd dump some into a pre-hab model, yet this just isn't part of professional sports yet. Instead, top trainers who know how to "condition an athlete" for a game are used—but the pre-hab aspect of sports conditioning is sadly overlooked.

The no-pain, no-gain psychology is truly a known component of athletic performance; having the psychology to endure pain is part of athleticism. You don't want your athletes whining about their body aching, and anyway, they believe it's *supposed* to ache because that's how they know they've worked hard enough. I've worked with professional athletes, so I know that their coaches aren't gung-ho about pre-hab, as many feel it alters the necessary psychology required to be an elite athlete. It's true that sports psychology plays a big factor in athletic performance; but trust me, athletes still get injured no matter how strong their belief is that they are impervious to pain.

This is the heart of the issue, and why MELT Performance is, literally, your very own version of pre-hab. We believe we are proactive on so many levels—but when it comes to stress injuries, we are *reactive*. We do things to *fix problems* far more than we do things *to avoid them.*

I had a driving passion to transform these powerful hands-on techniques into a "hands-off" method that my clients could use to improve their *own* stability and performance. MELT Performance is the culmination of decades of refinement and extraordinary results I've witnessed time and again in my private practice. Using the foundational concepts of manual muscle testing and hands-on neuromuscular reintegration techniques, I developed a few key techniques—Reintegrate and Repattern—and began sharing them with my clients. I taught them how to repeat these techniques at home between sessions to sustain the results they left my office with. It actually worked, except most of them stopped doing it once they started feeling good—which is why, over time, they needed to come back to see me.

I would ask them why, when they started having problems again, they didn't just go back and practice the Reintegrate and Repattern techniques I had already shown them. And they'd say that they had been feeling so good for so long, they had forgotten the moves. I heard this time and again in those days before the internet and easy digital access. Now my clients can go to MELT On Demand to watch videos and practice their techniques—empowering them to stay out of my office.

What was bothersome and perplexing to me was that despite many immediate and lasting changes in clients who had suffered a recent injury, the changes weren't as profound for clients with chronic pain or pain caused by surgery, medicine, or illness. I often felt that there was a bigger, underlying, unresolved issue as so many clients returned for a "tune-up" more frequently when a chronic issue had originally brought them to my practice.

I began experimenting with random tools to simulate hands-on techniques to see whether I could uncover the underlying issue and help my clients sustain changes far longer. I was motivated by a client who had come to me with neck pain, chronic migraines, and jaw pain after shoulder surgery. One day she said to me, "If you could just invent a way for me to do to myself what you do with your magic hands, I'd stay out of your office longer"—and I became determined to find a way for her to do just that. I made a soft roller by wrapping bubble wrap around PVC piping and then wrapping that in a yoga blanket and a yoga mat, and then duct-taping it all together. This tool gave just the right amount of compression, similar to what I accomplished with my forearm. I also bought every type of soft ball that was the approximate size of my elbow and thumb that my clients could use to simulate other hands-on techniques.

As I continued to experiment with these tools on my own body, as well as teaching my private clients how to do it at home between sessions, I witnessed profound changes. My clients would return with changes that I'd never seen before. And for myself, I found that I slept better and my neck and low back didn't crack or ache anymore. I didn't know it at the time, but as I continued to develop these techniques, I was building the foundations of the MELT Method.

▌ How Pain Transformed My Life

I worked my way through my undergrad and graduate programs as a competitive cyclist, fitness instructor, and personal trainer. My body fat was an astonishingly low 11 percent. I am only 5 feet, 6 inches tall, and at the time, I weighed 140 pounds. My arms were so big that people used to call me Guns. Or Diesel! I was at the peak of my fitness career. I had the body everybody said that they wanted. I was incredibly lean, and fit, and buff. I had the opportunity to appear on ESPN2's show *Crunch Fitness* and was the creator of the super-trendy *Boot Camp Training* video, which is still available online. I seemed to epitomize health and wellness, but I was in pain. Not a day went by that I wasn't achy, stiff, or hurting. I hid that from my clients. No pain, no gain, right? In fact, like many fitness professionals and athletes, I assumed that being achy and stiff was normal.

In the late 1990s, after nearly five years in clinical practice, I suffered an unusual pain in my body that I'd never experienced before. I'd had years of sprained ligaments, broken bones, and even a mild concussion, but this pain was different. It didn't come from a sudden identifiable trauma. I literally woke up one morning with a pain in the bottom of my foot that was so sharp I instantly thought, *I must have stepped on a piece of glass*. The pain persisted for weeks, leading to a dull ache in the back of my leg, then my low back, and then slowly moving up to my neck and jaw. After a few months, I started seeking help from my peers and mentors. I saw top doctors all over New York City who poked and prodded me to figure out what was going on and told me I had plantar fasciitis. It started to affect me not only on a structural level, but on a deep emotional level (see more in Chapter 3).

I very nearly lost my mind. I recall sitting on the cold tiles of my bathroom floor with a scalpel in my hand, ready to cut my foot open. What started out as plantar fasciitis had led to a body-wide ache, emotional depression, and a shift in my belief that neuromuscular therapy could fix anything—because no matter how much I tried to fix myself, nothing made a dent in the chronic pain I was now experiencing. I was witnessing my entire career and dreams go right down the toilet I was sitting next to.

This type of unrelenting, lingering pain is what I now define as a *sudden chronic pain*, meaning it comes on suddenly but is in fact caused by an accumulation of stuck stress. I'd done nothing out of the ordinary—I simply woke up one day with this new chronic pain. It was similar to the kind of athletic pain that suddenly occurs when you're doing a move or exercise you've done a thousand times before: You lean over to pick up a tennis ball, and your hamstring pulls. I hadn't sustained a traumatic event that caused sudden pain—it was literally an out-of-nowhere pain.

Two years after my foot pain first appeared, I had a newfound understanding of the importance of connective tissue, and my entire view of longevity and resilience completely shifted. By adding fascial therapy—a direct intervention that restores fluid flow to the connective tissue system—a true revelation occurred. My mind and body felt more grounded, and my connection to my movements and stability became ever present. My awareness and perspective of a stable body shifted. The power I gave to all of the musculoskeletal anatomy and physiology I'd spent more than a decade learning about suddenly took a backseat to the science I'd stumbled upon simply to find a solution to my own pain.

The years went by and I continued to develop ways to help my clients restore stability and balance back to their bodies, but then the horrible events of 9/11 occurred in my city. My overnight crash course in post-traumatic stress disorder (PTSD) would both challenge my beliefs in what causes pain to become chronic and deepen my understanding of how to shift the neurological pathways that cause pain to become chronic in the first place. Even when pain was chronic because of emotional trauma, MELT helped the neurological regulators of stress and repair balance again. Seeing how well this worked deepened my desire to help more diverse and challenging clients. It also made me realize just how much my personal history was a catalyst for my own chronic pain. I'm still astounded and gratified each time I help a person shift out of a downward spiral back into active living.

By 2004, I had coined the term M.E.L.T. Method, which stood for Myofascial Energetic Length Technique. By 2008, however, the acronym outgrew the method, so today I call it just MELT. It's the perfect word to describe how MELT allows you to return a stiff, inflexible body into a more fluid, flexible, and resilient form.

I started teaching group classes in the basic MELT protocols, and that's where the language of MELTing took shape. I began calling the moves and specific process Rehydrate techniques. I developed neck and low back decompression techniques I'd eventually call Release techniques. Then, as I refined my understanding of connective tissue's relationship to the involuntary aspects of our autonomic nervous system, I ultimately created *Rebalance* and *Reconnect* techniques. Those are the Four Rs of MELT.

My aha moment came when I realized how powerful connective tissue is when it comes to muscle timing and movement performance. By adding the Four Rs into the mix of my original NeuroStrength techniques, the most profound results I saw were that the reintegrative process to reacquire joint stability exponentially improved and the changes lasted far longer.

In my private practice I took copious notes and tracked my clients' progress. After their joints stopped hurting, they would keep MELTing at home because it felt good and made immediate changes. Once they did the basic MELT protocol, they had to do NeuroStrength only once or twice a week for ten to fifteen minutes to not only sustain changes, but to see changes in their performance.

That happened because these moves give the connective tissue the hydration it needs and also change how the brain's motor processing works. I had cracked the code. I realized that if you improve the body's natural stability by restoring the integrity of the connective tissue system, and *then* you reintegrate and repattern natural neurological function before you improve strength or mobility, your efforts work better and last a *lot* longer. As I integrated these techniques, the changes I witnessed took me by surprise. I'd never witnessed a group of people limp into my MELT class and walk out feeling stable and strong without my manually manipulating them at all. Hands-Off Bodywork became a real and powerful thing.

After this success in one-on-one and group settings, I began sharing these techniques with other practitioners so they too could help their clients even when those clients weren't in the office getting a massage, bodywork, or acupuncture session. Today, there are more than one thousand MELT classes and hundreds of MELT Performance classes taking place worldwide, taught by trained MELT instructors, to help people reverse and prevent pain and achieve new levels of performance. With this book, you can truly take your stability and performance to the next level without fear of damaging your joints through your training.

▶ MELT Performance Will Change Your Life

MELT Performance is the culmination of decades of refinement and extraordinary results. My focused techniques have helped me empower my clients to actively participate in restoring and sustaining ideal function even when doctors have told them that medication or surgery is their only option. I always say it's like fine-tuning an instrument. You must reacquire the proper tone, connection, vibration, and frequency of your body's connective tissue and your brain's neural pathways first, and then introduce new patterns.

I've lost count of the number of skeptics who told me that MELTing can't possibly work because it's too simple and easy to be true. But after they give in and try it, sure enough, they find that in just a matter of weeks they seem to move with greater ease and efficiency, their performance improves, and their energy increases.

As I edge toward my fifties, I can honestly say I look and feel better now than I did two decades ago when this journey started. With MELT Performance, my body is going to last the test of time. That bunion which wants to take over my foot and be crippling just like my mother's bunion? It hasn't gotten worse in twenty years, because I pay attention to it by doing the MELT Bunion Treatment. I fully plan to be as active and fit as I am now as I move through my fifties and into my sixties and beyond.

But the only way that will happen is to support the body's systems, which naturally break down and go south as we age. I'm going to be proactive and preventative, even though people constantly say, "But that maybe-bunion isn't bothering you. It hasn't changed. Why do you still bother with that bunion treatment?" Because, of course, that's precisely why that maybe-bunion is still a no-way-bunion! It's also why I still haven't had knee surgery despite a doctor telling me twenty-six years ago that the tears in my meniscus were so bad my only option was removing it. My knee never hurts, and although in the past I couldn't run because it hurt my knee or caused other pain, I now run several times every week with no pain or fear of injury.

With MELT Performance, you'll go into your body's basement and pour a new foundation. You will rewire your neurofascial system (nervous system + connective tissue system) so that you move the way you're supposed to move and connect to your body in a totally new way. This book will show you how to properly set up and execute each move so you get the same results you would get if you had a private session with me, saving you time and money while empowering you to live an active, healthy, pain-free life.

For those of you who are already avid MELTers, MELT Performance will make MELTing work even better. You will learn some of the most forward-thinking concepts about connective tissue, neurological stability, and sensorimotor control. From my perspective, our economy and Big Pharma outweigh all of the progressive and obvious advancements we can harness to improve our health. Updating medical and college textbooks, modernizing surgical methods, and expanding the education of doctors beyond medical school seems improbable. It's as if health care has become a sick care industry. Doctors don't practice prevention. They practice cure. Ideally, the only time you really need a doctor is when you are looking to cure a problem that you can't fix yourself. Preventing your need to go to the doctor means learning that the best health care is self-care. That's what MELT is all about. Self-care is the best care.

My learning is constant, often overwhelming, but my curiosity and passion to learn about longevity, aging, and the pursuit of happiness and good health leave me wanting to know more and share everything I discover. In the early 1900s Thomas Edison said, "The doctor of the future will give no medicine but will interest his patients in the care of the human frame, in diet and in the cause and prevention of disease." We all have within us an inner warrior, an inner athlete awaiting the next challenge life brings. I hope MELT Performance brings yours to the forefront to express its strength, allowing you to crush every goal you want to reach.

But more than anything, I hope you recognize that your body is filled with a strength and power that are beyond muscle strength and power; that you can reclaim your body's natural resilience, a piece of your life; that you can embrace and empower it in love that is far deeper and more important than the muscle part of you. It's time to seize the initiative and make your body function better. I'm asking you to commit and be *proactive* about your health instead of *reactive* to injuries and illness. I'm asking you to go for the little bit of change and realize that it's not going to be painful. In fact, it's empowering.

And the really good news is that what I'm asking you to incorporate into your life only takes a few minutes a day—but it will leak into every facet of your life. You're going to start thinking differently about movement, exercise, performance, and life itself. You're going to transform your whole body and your whole life, for years to come.

MELT Performance will transform your body, mind, and spirit from the inside out. There will never be a day in your life when you can't MELT!

So what are you waiting for? Let's go!

PART ONE

Creating NeuroStrength

1

Defining NeuroStrength and Redefining Stability

When I made my first presentation about connective tissue at the IDEA Fitness Conference in 2003, someone said to me: "I don't get how this has anything to do with fitness. This has nothing to do with how to make my body leaner and fitter."

"It *does* have to do with fitness," I replied. "In fact, it's more important than being lean and fit, because it's about your overall resilience, longevity, and ability to sustain optimal performance today and even when you're old. You're more likely to get injured trying to get lean and fit than working at a desk all day. It's the dirty little secret of fitness—most of the people in the gym are managing aches and pain and frequently lose all their short-term gains because of stress injuries. So this has everything to do with fitness."

That person shrugged. "I don't get it. You can't exercise your fascia."

So there I was, frustrated that all this amazing information I'd been amassing wasn't reaching its audience. I soon realized, however, that talking about connective tissue *on a microscopic level* didn't make sense to fitness professionals because their training has nothing to do with this. But this was where the information needed to be, and I decided to translate these concepts so more people could learn how to live a better life. People who know me know that I'm not a fitness guru, but I am a geek who loves research and applying science to everyday life. My passion is sharing this information with anyone looking to improve performance, decrease their risk of injuries, and reduce chronic aches and accumulated stress so they don't impede their ability to feel great today and tomorrow.

As I changed my wording, I inadvertently created a simplified language—what I call the Living Body Model—to explain the importance of connective tissue and the nervous system to every aspect of a person's overall heath.

When I first started sharing MELT in group environments, I talked a lot about connective tissue dehydration. I even brought strips of cow fascia into my class to help me explain why this tissue is so unique. But then a guy in class said, "Sue, I don't really know what connective tissue is."

That's when the light bulb went off. "Do you ever find that when you move out of a position, like going from sitting to standing, some of your joints ache?" I asked.

"All the time," he said with a chuckle.

"Well, think of connective tissue like a sponge. Have you ever woken up feeling as stiff as a sponge left out overnight on your kitchen sink? Daily living decreases the moist, fluid state of connective tissue. It gets dehydrated on a cellular level, and then it doesn't adapt as fast as it should. Now your joints are full of stuck stress altering your ability to move efficiently."

"I *am* full of stuck stress," he agreed.

When it comes to stability and control, people actually *think* they know a lot about those topics, yet most people are actually acquiring stability and control in a faulty way, because stability and control are all based within our *neurofascial system* (the system that connects the fascial and nervous systems), meaning it's involuntary in the first place—so the crazy thing is, we don't know that any of this is happening. Even athletes and people who do everything right still accumulate stress in their bodies, in a way that compromises the stability of their joints.

This chapter teaches you about neurological stability, or *NeuroStrength.* NeuroStrength will save your joints unnecessary tension, compression, and misalignment, and you will improve your muscular timing and overall motor control—the true foundation of power, agility, and strength.

In *The MELT Method*, I focused on reconnecting you to your body so you could identify stuck stress and common imbalances before they cause you pain. With MELT Performance, we'll take all of this a step farther and harness the power of your neurological stability system. You will learn how to rewire your neural pathways of stability to improve function. In the scientific community, we know that neurons that "fire together, wire together"; if the wiring is faulty, we now know that we can rewire the faulty pathways and rebuild them.

When you have neurological stability, you don't think about having it or how you move. You simply move in the way you're meant to. If someone in another room asks me to come see something, for example, I instantly get up and go have a look. That is a healthy, normal response. But if someone asks the same of my mother, she won't get up from the chair where she spends most of her time. Instead, she says, "Can't you come here?" Her brain is actively trying to figure out how to do what it is asked to do without actually having to do it. Her primal, foundational stability and control system is faulty.

MELT Performance will undo your own faulty patterns and give you a new, sturdy, stable foundation.

- STEP 1: You create the environment for your nervous system to function more efficiently and for stability to exist by MELTing and hydrating your connective tissue.

- STEP 2: You then reintegrate neurological joint stability and control. The setup of the moves is the key to unlocking this potential.

- STEP 3: You repattern your basic motor patterns. This way your movements are more efficient, effortless, and accessible in everyday living.

MELT Performance takes only a few minutes a day and allows you to quickly adapt. You can hop over a cat sitting in the hallway or dodge a child learning how to ride a bike. You can jump up onto a sidewalk. You can get out of the way of a moving car. All without even thinking about it. You will create resilience in your body.

This really is a game-changer. Like most people, I believed that eating right and exercising regularly would allow me to lead a more active and healthy life. Don't get me wrong, these *are* essential elements of a healthy life. But if that were all it took to lead a pain-free, active life, then everyone who engages in fitness would be free of pain. But they aren't, of course—like I said, it's a dirty little secret of the fitness industry that people who train to be fit and healthy are the ones most frequently trying to resolve pain in their bodies. Because fitness professionals and enthusiasts become so obsessed with training their muscles to improve the tone, shape, and size of their bodies, they forget that their *joints* are more critical than their muscle strength. I've heard of people getting knee and hip replacements, but I've never heard of someone getting a hamstring replacement.

▶ Why Reestablishing Joint Stability Is So Important

Most people don't know they have faulty habits and compensation that lead them to damage their bodies despite their own efforts and desire to stay healthy. The NeuroStrength you'll develop with MELT Performance will stop that process from happening. It will instead keep your body supple and resilient and improve joint stability, motor control, and muscle timing. You'll be able to restore primary neurological pathways of stability and get your body's stability mechanisms back on track.

The reason why? Reestablishing joint stability is the key to maximizing potential and performance and decreasing your risk of injuries. Professional athletes and their trainers don't realize that even when they have great muscle strength, their neurological stability is often weak, which can leave them feeling like they have to train even harder. All athletes hit a plateau in their training, and often their psychological mindset makes them try to run faster, hit a ball harder, or deadlift a heavier weight to try to hoist themselves out of that state. Many people who want to become great athletes are told to push themselves—but all too often, this push can send them over the edge, causing long-term issues that could have been avoided.

I saw this all the time in my neuromuscular therapy practice. When I started, I mostly worked with athletes who had gotten injured playing their sport and were seeking help to get back at it. During my initial evaluation of their alignment, movement, and injury, I often found imbalances in other regions of their body that were the real cause of their repeated injuries or why they weren't recovering fully.

The reality is, athletes are compensating machines and don't know it. Their body's amazing adaptability to their repetitive training routines is often the reason they get injured in the first place. Despite how much agility, strength, and power they seem to possess, their ability to harness these aspects are hindered because of a loss in joint stability and control.

The notion of neurological instability was hard for these athletes to wrap their brains around. They *felt* strong, but neurologically, their brains and bodies weren't communicating efficiently. What was easy for them to recognize was that the goals they used to easily achieve now required more effort and energy.

These athletes didn't yet realize that it was the *compensation* they'd been engaging in for years that was causing their stress injuries and setting them up for repeated injuries in the future. Remember that these people were super-strong and fit and often very flexible. They knew their bodies inside and out (or at least they thought they did!). The issue wasn't their muscles giving them pain, but the neurological mechanisms that were no longer giving them the joint stability and range of motion they needed. The protective mechanisms of the body are profound, and the compensation to preserve them had actually started working against the gains that these athletes wanted to make.

For example, if your hamstrings are locked short and tight, you instinctively think the best thing to do is to stretch them. What you may not realize is that tight hamstrings can be your body's protective means to support the sacroiliac (SI) joints in your pelvis. Shortening the hamstring will decrease the axis of rotation the SI joints possess to allow us to walk with ease. In this case, it's as if the smoke detector is going off to alert you that your toaster's on fire—yet your response is to take the batteries out of the smoke detector to stop it from beeping. The alarm is now off, but the toaster is still burning. Stretching out your hamstrings won't change the fact that your SI joint is still compromised. You just took away the alert and the protection, so not only have you increased your chances of a more catastrophic injury, but you can get real damage that you can't stretch your way out of.

My injured athletic clients needed to stop thinking about their muscles as a means of recovery and to work on the neurological stability of their joints instead. Traditional exercise protocols, sports-specific training, and even physical therapy didn't cut it. What also clicked is when I told them to think about their bodies as if they were buildings constructed atop rollers to prevent earthquake damage. Even the most durable skyscraper can crack and topple when the earth moves—but it won't if it has built-in elasticity and adaptability that allow it to sway and reduce its stress load and transmit force to all of the components of the building in the worst-case scenario. A human body with neurological stability has that same kind of fluidity, and our fascia is that elastic, adaptable environment we need to harness.

◗ How Fascia Affects Your Functions

Before we get into neurological joint stability, it's very important to know what connective tissue is and does, because giving this amazing substance the attention it needs is what activates the potential to restore neurological stabilization.

When we think of anatomy, we tend to think about muscles and bones, with perhaps a few tendons or ligaments thrown in. We all want nice firm arms and strong legs, and we want to be able to run fast and push hard if we're so inclined. But the leverage that you're producing to push yourself doesn't come from your muscles alone. It comes through the whole connective tissue system that's everywhere, from your skin all the way to your bones. If you deplete it, if you don't replenish it, if you don't care for it, you're going to be the athlete or the person who gets sick, who gets hurt, whose repetition catches up to them and leads to stress injuries. Who ages poorly. Who feels crummy all the time. Who looks dull and blah. Who gets grumpy. Who's unhappy. And who never gets ahead in life. That's not going to be you anymore, right?

Fascia is your body's three-dimensional, embryological, anatomical, fluid-based support system; it's an interwoven, head-to-toe network that gives you stability and protection. There's no discontinuity in the layers of fascia, although the word *layers* may be deceptive. While the molecular components are continuous, certain regions can be defined and are called *layers* or *sheaths*.

Think of your fascia like the elements of an orange—after you peel the fruit, you see the white pith around the exterior; go deeper and you see that the orange is divided into segments; go deeper still and you see that each bit of pulp is also surrounded by a membrane. No matter how small the division, it's all part of the same system.

You don't need to understand fascia scientifically to give it the attention it needs, but I think what science has learned about fascia is fascinating. Fascia is a tissue devised of tiny compartments and fibers, made from countless micro-fibrils (liquid-lined fibers, like straws) that form the collagen network, and multi-microvacuolar spaces that hold vital fluids (like water and other gel-like substances called glycosaminoglycans, or GAGs, and hyaluronan). These amazing collagen fibrils can change and adapt—anticipating your movements as they lengthen or shorten, kind of like bendy straws. These elements are manufactured by the various fascial cells as they continuously monitor and fix the fascial environment so it remains stable in all directions.

The definition of fascia has recently expanded to include the cells that create and maintain the extracellular matrix (ECM). *Extracellular matrix* isn't an interchangeable term for *fascia*, by the way. The extracellular matrix refers to everything outside the cells, whereas the fascia includes the cells that produce, maintain, and break down the ECM. Fascia is the link between the ECM and all other definable elements in your body.

I go into more detail about the developments in research in Chapter 4, but for now what's important to understand is that the building materials—the fibers, gels, and water content—of the ECM are everywhere and that this connective tissue is called fascia.

When stress is applied, the tissues adapt—for better or worse. For example, fascial adaptability helps us enhance our skill to throw a ball with speed and accuracy as the tissue anticipates how we want to move. It's also what helps you keep your head forward while working at your desk, but when you get up and move around, that tissue adaptation keeps your head fixed in that position even when you don't want or need it there. Although genetics plays a role in determining what proteins are manufactured (a key cause of many connective tissue disorders), our daily living and how we use our body determine how our tissues adapt. Fascia disperses force throughout all of its components to manage our movements as best as it can, and repetition can both help and hinder this management.

Fascia is also an information highway that supports all aspects and systems of your body. Loaded with sensory nerve endings, fascia is like an antenna, pulling in signals and sending out information.

As I wrote in *The MELT Method*, my understanding of fascia completely changed under the tutelage of Gil Hedley, who teaches courses on integral anatomy and dissection. I learned that, contrary to what is taught in medical school and anatomy textbooks, fascia is far more than just an inert packing material. During the many dissections I did with Gil, I learned how to uncover fascia's many layers, which piqued my curiosity to find others who view fascia as an important component of our well-being.

Gil upended everything I thought I knew about fascia. As I searched for more research, I went down a deep rabbit hole of molecular, neurological, cellular, and non-cellular science. I began to understand why our nervous system is not just some independent thing that is in charge of directing all bodily functions. Instead, our nervous system—our neurological functioning—relies on fascia, the environment it lives in, to function efficiently. Further, fascia interconnects with all our other cells, allowing them to communicate with each other so they too can function properly.

In other words, fascia has a link to neurological stability. The sudden chronic foot pain I had at the peak of my fitness career wasn't pain caused by an injury. No orthopedist knew how to fix it—because that injury wasn't in my muscles or bones. My condition also led me to understand how fascia plays a role in our emotional stability. Figuring out how to heal my own sudden chronic pain drove me to understand the link between muscles, bones, nerves, blood vessels, organs, and even emotions.

Fascia is the only system in the body that isn't dependent on the nervous system. It can morph and adapt, and it does this independently of neurological response or activation. But fascia needs to be healthy and supple—what I call hydrated—in order to function properly. When it isn't, it becomes less adaptable and less stable, and this affects how we function.

Your fascia is also designed to store energy so that whatever you do, you do it really well for long periods of time. If you want your body to sit because you have to be at your desk for most of the day, your fascia is going to adapt so that you can hold that posture without using unnecessary energy. That's great, in theory, but human beings are not designed to sit still for long periods. Even though the modern world has accelerated, allowing us to gain everything from information to lunch without moving at all, we aren't very far off from our cave-dwelling ancestors, genetically speaking, and we're still driven by the fight-or-flight response when stressed.

This is why MELT Performance is so important: It allows you to focus on and care for your fascial and nervous systems and strive for improved stability so that you move better. Far beyond muscle strength, NeuroStrength will help you learn more about how your fascia affects neurological control, efficiency, and overall stability. It will help you train smarter and take you to a higher level of performance without training harder.

▶ Defining NeuroStrength

How does the nervous system work? Scientists have yet to crack the code, because the majority of our body's functions are *autonomic*, meaning involuntary and out of our conscious control. So when people say, "I am in control of me," I think, "Well, you are in charge of maybe 3 percent of you, because 97 percent of your body's physical functions are done without your thinking about it." That's the problem with pain—it's subjective, meaning that a person's perception of pain overrides objective findings. Here's a simple example: If I punch two people in the arm with the same amount of pressure, one might fall to the ground and tell me they're going to sue me for damages, and the other might simply laugh or punch me back. There's a *lot* of subjective reasoning behind both reactions, and neither may have a thing to do with what the person actually felt in the moment. Rather, it's the history and memories of being hit or punched that make them respond the way they do. I know this might sound complex, but as the next two chapters unfold, you'll better understand and relate to this idea of how we perceive control, balance, and pain.

Your ability to function relies on your autonomic responses—from breathing to digesting food to sleeping through the night. I call the system responsible for these functions your Autopilot. Imagine if you had to think about breathing, or you had to will your heart to beat. You'd frequently pass out, and sleeping would be out of the question. At the very least, you'd never be able to do anything except focus on the basic functions that keep you alive—to the detriment of everything else. The concept of fear would take on a whole new meaning.

A lot of your daily activities happen without your conscious awareness. For example, when you tie your shoes or walk across the street, are you *really* thinking about what you're doing? You just do it. Patterns become habit; habits becomes gesture; gestures becomes form and function. Your Autopilot is in control of all that as it goes through its daily tasks of constant compensation and adaptation to whatever situation or environment it's in.

Notice that I'm not using the word *brain.* The brain, although an important part of the nervous system, is just a *part* of that system. Even the brain has subsystems that most people don't know much about. Beyond the tissue that comprises the many definable regions of the brain, both neuron cell bodies and non-neuron brain cells called glial cells play body-wide roles in our overall well-being and function. The nervous system is far more complex than just the tissue we define as the brain. It's a whole-body, integrated system with one primary job: to keep us alive and moving. That's a big job. What perplexes science is how our nervous system can go haywire and work against our proper cell development and overall health. The nervous system is far more complex than a computer, but modern-day technology is allowing us to understand and measure aspects of the nervous system in new ways. In just the past fifty years, we've learned more about the nervous system than ever before.

If we knew everything we could about the brain's potential to uptake information, process it, and then use it, we'd be able to stop in their tracks Alzheimer's disease, Parkinson's disease, multiple sclerosis, epilepsy, dementia, bipolar disorder, depression, and all other brain and nervous system conditions. Motor control, movement, and how the nervous system allows our body to perform many tasks without our thinking about them are multifaceted processes that are hard to define. Yet the nervous system is malleable, pliable, and adaptable. It is able to make new neural connections every minute of every day, no matter how old we are. This is what makes NeuroStrength such a powerful practice.

You don't need a lot of intricate products, tools, or time to continue learning and making new neuronal connections—you just need to understand the what, how, and why of neurological reintegration. These three components are all it takes to understand what's missing currently in your wellness and fitness protocols and to be able to implement the moves and sequences you'll learn about in Part Two of this book to achieve the outcomes that traditional training regimens often miss.

▶ The Science of Stability

The human body has a hardwired, innate need to maintain balance. This is what science calls homeostasis. On every level—emotional, chemical, and structural—our body is constantly adapting, shifting, and interpreting both the internal and external environments to maintain the balance it needs to keep itself alive. When we run, for example, our body cools us by sweating. When we eat food, our body secretes enzymes to break down the nutrients we ingest.

When you think of a body that is unstable, what image do you see? I'll bet you imagine an older person with a walker or someone with a limp. Or maybe someone with a disability or brain disease. These can indeed be considered examples of instability, but they are on the far end of the instability spectrum.

Stability is actually not what you think. The stability that counts is not based on muscular strength or motor control. Rather, it's *structural strength* that's important. Structural strength is the capacity of individual elements to withstand load and transmit forces from gravity to movement to all the elements within a structure. If our structural strength is out of balance, joints pay the price. People can do a lot of movements poorly, and again, they don't even know that on a functional or structural level their exercise choices are often doing more harm than good when it comes to their joints. Even people who look perfect performing an exercise or a training drill may have neurological instability and are compensating to do what looks so perfect. They can become what I call segmentally flexible or segmentally strong—which is to say, parts of their body move too much and become hypermobile, and in other areas the muscles are locked short and move too little, causing joints to compress. Either way, instability ensues, and their chances of injury vastly increase over time.

When I say "stability," I'm not talking about how well you balance or how aligned your posture looks when you stand up. Instead, I'm talking about neurological stability and how you produce movement patterns. What you think is strong and stable might not be.

Neurological Stability

Neurological stability is your nervous system being able to stabilize your joints before you even move. Hydrated fascia allows force to be transmitted beyond the linear muscle-to-tendon direction so that no single joint endures the full weight or stress of any motion. In general, when fascia is hydrated and the nervous system is working efficiently, stability is completely *involuntary*.

Every joint has an amount of motion that is natural for it, which is why your range of motion may be quite different from someone else's. In addition, stability is not about how much movement you have (quantity) but rather about how well you can control it (quality and accuracy).

So whenever I use the word *stability*, don't think about your muscles, or standing on an uneven surface and trying to balance. Instead, think about whether your body can respond quickly to remain stable in all directions and move efficiently from day to day.

To achieve this, you need an orchestration of what I call neurofascial communication. The two primary systems of our body that provide support, connection, stability, and control are our nervous system and our connective tissue system. Together, the neurofascial system—our Autopilot—is responsible for keeping us relatively upright, stable, and functioning as efficiently as possible.

This is how I explained the concept of the Autopilot and stability to a newbie in one of my classes: "Okay," I told him, "you've got a whole bunch of stuck stress in your body, which is limiting your movement and making you feel stiff and un-stable. Your body is stronger, yet more dysfunctional. You're like a compensating machine—your body's nervous system has learned to manage your instability better, but you aren't actually improving your joint stability because your basic workouts don't address the problem. That's why your back and knees always ache. You're compensating just to pick up your water bottle from the floor, and you don't even know that's happening. Does that make sense?"

He nodded. "But what about that neuro thing you keep mentioning?"

"Neurological stability and regulation. Well, when it comes to stability and neuro-logical regulation, we don't really think about how that works. We don't think about stability at all, in fact. We don't even think about moving—we just move."

I told him to think about his body like the autopilot in an airplane. Aside from taking off and landing the plane, the autopilot does basically everything to sustain the plane in the air. Unless a blinking red light goes off to alert the pilot that something's not right, the pilot just enjoys the ride. That's what we do, too, with our bodies. We don't bother to recognize the subtle signs of instability and dysfunction in our bodies because there are no blinking lights. The pre-pain signs that our Autopilot creates, like feeling stiff when we get up out of a chair after sitting for a period of time, are such common sensations that we think they're normal, so we never do anything about them. We're like the pilot who waits until the plane's engines aren't firing and the plane's in a downward spiral with loud alarms going off before taking over the controls and trying to save the plane from crashing and burning.

The problem with these two involuntary and powerful global systems is that often their way of keeping us stable over time compromises our overall well-being. The nervous system isn't doing this on purpose; it's just how it and our connective tissue system work.

For example, if you don't eat very well and don't sleep well, but you go for a run anyway, you're challenging your neurofascial system to function with efficiency. To remain efficient and get the job done, first it will slow down any unnecessary processes it's responsible for. You get symptoms that you either brush off or don't notice—again, those are pre-pain signals. Your back and neck will always be a little stiff or tight, and you'll be aware of it when you stand up from a sitting position. Your hair and skin are always dry. Your muscles take longer to repair so you feel achy many days after you work out. You don't realize it, but these systems are altering your stress, repair, metabolic, and digestive regulators to keep the important components of your body working well enough for you to keep going. I always think of this like your computer working in safety or energy-efficient mode, or setting your phone to airplane mode to save battery power.

The Difference Between Muscle Strength and Structural Strength

Despite the power of the six-hundred-plus muscles in your body, strong muscles are *not* what stabilize your joints. You can be as strong as an ox and able to bench-press your weight twenty times, but this doesn't mean that you're not going to have back pain. In fact, doing this kind of weight lifting without joint stability will guarantee that you *will* have pain!

At the peak of my fitness career, my muscles were so huge and shaped so distinctively into very firm and well-defined V's, especially on my back and shoulders, that I was often asked whether I was a competitive swimmer. I was fit and lean and looked amazing. Yet these muscles I worked so hard to bulk up were literally crushing my bone structure. I didn't know at the time that what stabilizes the joints is not the strength of muscles, but connective tissue, bones, and muscles working seamlessly together, feeding each other good synergy, good timing, and good motor control. I didn't need to be muscularly stronger—I needed to be more *structurally stable*. I had to rethink what true stability is.

Once I realized how important it is to treat your connective tissue *first* and then reintegrate and repattern your neural connections, I was able to help my body move in the way that it was designed to move, not in the way that we've programmed it to because of our modern lifestyles. No matter how strong your muscles are, if you sit all day, you're altering the structure of your body, and your muscles start a compensation cascade. Your joints pay the price. Your body misaligns. You start to hurt. You increase inflammation. You pop an ibuprofen, you start over, but your joints don't get a break.

In recent times, scientists have taken to using the term *biotensegrity*. The architectural term *tensegrity* (a word made by blending the words *tension* and *integrity*) defines a structure that is stable in three dimensions and disperses force throughout the entire structure so no one element has to manage the demand of tension or compression forces. The integrity of the rigging is what holds the struts in the right place. In a human body, bones are struts, and muscles are movers leveraging the bones so we can move; but the collagen matrix, our fascia, that holds them and keeps them floating in a stable environment are like tiny strong wires managing force and sustaining our architectural stability. Knowing how to improve the collagen matrix and its supportive qualities is missing in most athletic programs.

▶ Self-Assess and Self-Reassess for NeuroStrength

In working with high-performance athletes, I learned early on that their belief system and mindset were pretty hardwired. Forget reality—if they *believed* they were stable, my trying to persuade them that neurological instability was the cause of their stress injury was not easy. My ability to test them didn't really convince them, so self-assessment became necessary. Trying to explain what neurological stability is or how postural reflexes work was too complex, but having the athletes test their neurological stability, control, and accuracy themselves was easy to do and quickly made them realize that I knew something they didn't know. "Why didn't my coach tell me this was happening?" most of them asked me. My simple reply: "Your coach knows how to train you to be a better athlete and probably doesn't know what neurological stability is."

An essential part of MELT Performance are the self-assess and self-reassess phases. Self-assessing instability does a number of powerful things. First, it gives you a body baseline to work from. It also lets you quickly identify whether your self-care protocol is working and to value the changes you make for yourself. On a more profound level, it allows your nervous system to adapt more quickly to changes and sustain changes longer, thus improving your body baseline over time.

This was a big turning point in my understanding of the nervous system as well as empowering people to engage in and adopt a true self-care practice. Often, when a person is in chronic pain or has sought out a solution but gotten no results, what I call a *thought virus* is created—that is, the belief that nothing is going to help them, something really wrong is happening, and they can't fix the issue no matter how hard they try. These thoughts can shape the future before it happens and stop people from harnessing their true potential.

Simple Ways to Test and Assess Your Neurological Connection and Control

Let's test your neurological stability, control, and whole-body connection to see whether you have stuck stress limiting your overall functionality.

Reach and Touch Test

Stand up straight with bare feet. Reach your left arm over your head with your index finger pointed to the sky. Close your eyes and then reach up with your right arm and touch the tip of your left finger. Feel free to repeat this test on the other side.

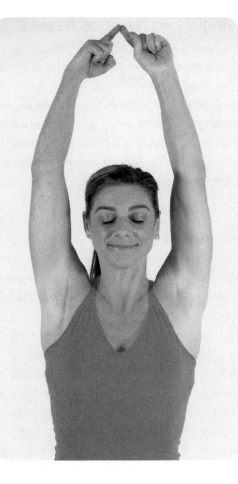

When you reached up, were you able to easily find the tip of your finger, or did you miss it or end up touching the middle of your finger? If you missed it, you are now learning what neurological inefficiency feels like. Your finger is attached to you. Why can't you find it when you reach up to it?

Think of your joints like satellites. Your nervous system is trying to identify where your joints are in relation to gravity, the ground, and your pelvis. Stuck stress, or connective tissue dehydration, can cause your brain to lose satellite reception in one or more joints. This is why your accuracy and control are less than perfect when you try to touch one of your extremities.

Single Leg Balance Assess

Stand tall with your feet hip-width apart, in bare feet, toes pointed straight ahead. Soften your left knee slightly to reduce hyperextension, bracing, or locking out your knee joint to increase your stability (no cheating!). Then, without shifting too far to the left, slowly lift your right leg and hold this single-leg stance for 30 seconds. Repeat on the other side.

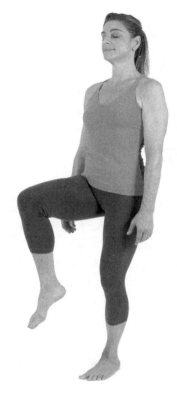

This is another simple way to test neurological efficiency and general balance and motor coordination. If you find that regardless of which leg you lift, you slightly tip or shift to a side, that's an indication that stability is being achieved in an inefficient way.

Next, repeat this same single-leg balance assessment, but once you lift one foot off the ground and you have found your balance, close your eyes. See if you can remain standing upright for at least fifteen seconds. Repeat on the other side.

This challenges your Autopilot (remember: the aspects of your neurofascial system that ideally support, protect, and stabilize you without your voluntary control or awareness) to go into action quickly and efficiently. If the stability mechanisms are faulty, you won't be able to remain upright and stable.

If you find in both assessments that you list, shift, or have to put one foot on the floor, you have found neurological instability. Most often, the side you tip to is the weaker side neurologically (not necessarily muscularly). Beyond muscle strength, when the timing of pelvic or shoulder stabilizers is faulty, your ability to remain upright on one foot is compromised. (Later, I'll teach you how to restore pelvic stability and the neurological mechanisms that control pelvic balance.)

In Chapter 5, I'll share another assessment to help you identify where stuck stress has accumulated throughout your body so you can eliminate it before you reintegrate neurological stability or repattern the stabilizers of your pelvis or shoulder girdle.

About Proprioception (Body Sense) and Your Muscles

Proprioception is your remarkable ability to know the exact position of your body in space and to react to your environment in a way that allows you to maintain your upright stance. It's also how you can instantly figure out where your nose is if you close your eyes and try to touch it. Some scientists call it the sixth sense.

An easy way to see whether your proprioception, or what I call Body Sense, is in good working order is with these easy self-assess tests: You should be able to freely stand on one leg, not holding onto anything for balance, with your eyes open for at least thirty seconds or with your eyes closed for fifteen seconds. This shows adequate mind-body communication—essential for those of us wanting to function efficiently in any sport or dynamic movement.

For proprioception, our neurofascial system uses specialized sensory nerve endings called proprioceptors and mechanoreceptors to send and receive information throughout the body. These receptors are found in high numbers within our joints. Most of them are in our hands, feet, and spine—the regions where we have more joints per square inch of our body.

The way we stabilize our pelvis, for example, comes partly from this proprioceptive system. Our body has more than six hundred muscles that are stimulated to contract by electrical signals from the nervous system. Muscles that are large and superficial, such as the gluteus maximus in our buttocks, have a primary job to move us. These are often called phasic muscles. Phasic muscles are composed of at least 51 percent fast-twitch muscle fibers. They are powerful muscles, but they fatigue more easily than the tonic muscles also known as stabilizers.

Muscles designed to stabilize local joints are often called local, postural, tonic, or core muscles. These muscles are primarily small, deep muscles that do not cause large movements, but they are positioned well for stabilizing the joints and do so without our conscious control. They are in fact always reacting and responding, independent of actual gross movement created when we act upon a stimulus. Tonic muscles are slow-twitch dominant, composed of at least 51 percent slow-twitch muscle fibers. As such, they are highly resistant to fatigue and have a greater propensity for work. The iliopsoas is an example of a tonic muscle group.

The greatest difference between phasic and tonic muscles is how these muscles and their fascial connections respond to tension, compression, or loading. This faulty loading occurs from repetition in the form of overuse, misuse, underuse, abuse, or simply aging.

What's interesting is that tonic muscles have a higher tendency to decrease our ability to move with ease. Even though their job isn't to actually move us, if they can't sustain joint position and stabilize a joint before movement, joint compression or excess tension can occur, causing pain. This causes our movers to be activated to stabilize a joint—so when we move, they aren't as efficient because they are already doing something. This causes muscles to become chronically short, tight, elongated, weak, or unable to activate. We feel this issue as pain or stiffness when we move. The more we repeat a movement or posture, the more the neurological stabilizing mechanisms are challenged to react and respond. The end result is compensation—we still move, but not efficiently.

As we age, these proprioceptors and our Body Sense decline, which is why so many older people lose their balance and fall more easily than they did when they were younger. If proprioception declines, our neurological connection to our pelvic position is hindered and makes us unstable on our feet.

▶ Establishing a NeuroStrength Foundation

Why is it so important to pour ourselves a new foundation now, even if we're strong, healthy, and fit? Because we learn how to be stable from the time we're infants, and if our foundation is faulty, then it becomes even more faulty with each passing year. From conception to death, structure begets function and function begets structure— an inevitable cycle of dysfunction that is bound to happen with our modern lifestyles.

The three key factors are:

- Primal patterns are established during infancy.

- When patterns become faulty, compensation takes over.

- Compensation is exacerbated by repetition of faulty patterns.

We Learn Stability from an Early Age

From conception through infancy, our body-mind connection and learning develop at the fastest pace they ever will. Newborns go from being helpless to crawling in a scant few months. Before you know it, they're pulling themselves up, then cruising between chairs and the sofa, and then standing fully upright and walking. Everything they're learning is brand new. After all, we only do everything for the first time once! If you have a baby, you've seen the excitement on that baby's face when he or she finds a foot or feels grass for the first time.

All babies are genetically programmed to develop reflexes that turn into notable milestones and markers that allow the neurons in their brains to fire together, wire together, and lay the foundation for their bodies to be able to move effectively and efficiently without thought. The seemingly haphazard motions a baby performs in the womb and continues to perform through the developmental phases after birth create the superhighways that the nervous system will ultimately use for all deliberate movement for the rest of the baby's life. These superhighways are called neural pathways, and they connect relatively distant areas of the brain or peripheral nervous system to each other.

Neurons, neural pathways, synapses, and brain plasticity are key factors in early brain development. The new field of epigenetics further confirms that environmental factors and nurturing during the early stages of life influence gene function throughout life. A baby being deprived of touch and loving experiences during the early years can have catastrophically negative effects on how some genes work, decreasing everything from basic intelligence to stress management as that baby grows.

In my years working with high-achieving athletes, I often asked them why they thought they had gotten to such a high level of skill. Most skirted around the answer, but ultimately many realized that, if they were praised and acknowledged when they hit a home run or won a race when they were young, they were more likely to try harder to reach even bigger achievements to acquire more praise.

Primal Patterns

No one teaches a baby how to walk, just as no mama bird teaches her nestlings how to fly. Animals are genetically programmed to move, and they just keep trying until the goal is reached. For human babies striving to get upright, the ultimate goal is to "get that thing," whether the thing is their primary parent or a tempting, shiny object. To do this, they must have a clear connection to their center of gravity—their pelvis—in an upright position. When they're still crawling, the center of gravity is relative to the navel. Before they even crawl, a baby's straight spine has to develop its curves to stabilize a large head over a small and unstable space called the neck. Then, to come up to a quadruped posture on all fours, they arch and do belly training; they reach out their arms and legs like Superman flying to engage the spinal extensors, allowing them to rock and ultimately move forward and backward.

If you think about your body, your head is far larger and heavier than your feet, and for babies, the head is often heavier than the rib region. How does their little body support that heavy head? Through neurological reflexes and mechanisms of stability.

Within these neural pathways are the primitive reflexes, righting reactions, equilibrium responses, and neurological mechanisms that we use to ultimately move efficiently in an upright posture. Primitive reflexes are basic movement patterns we create in response to repeated stimuli. When a mom reaches her arms out to her baby, the baby repeats the same movement pattern with little to no variation. Some of these primitive reflexes develop in utero and appear at or before birth! The postural reactions and movement responses to maintain balance develop later in infancy. As gravity becomes a stimulus to an infant, other reactions and responses develop that carry on through that infant's life.

The stage between crawling and walking, or cruising, is usually overlooked, but it's a very important transition from quadruped to standing and walking on two feet. While cruising, infants discover ways to control the torso in an upright position. They develop their primary motor programs. By the end of the cruising phase, infants are functionally quite skillful, but they continue to use multiple and varied patterns of control for a single task. They have learned to limit the degrees of freedom just enough to successfully accomplish the task at hand and, again, to ultimately "get that thing"—the shiny object or Mom or Dad.

By the time you were the age of two, these reflexes and mechanisms were hardwired into your body. If nothing got in the way of your properly developing these reflexes, reactions, and mechanisms of stability, you now have NeuroStrength. Your body integrates these pathways as the six primary functional motor patterns that together create the dynamic motions and functional patterns we take for granted, such as the basic walking pattern called gait. These functional motor patterns are:

- *Flexion:* The action of bending, or a movement that decreases the angle between two body parts.

- *Extension:* The opposite of flexion, or the straightening movement that increases the angle between body parts. Both flexion and extension are movements that occur in the sagittal plane or forward and backward motions.

- *Rotation:* A movement where part of your body pivots or revolves around the long axis. Medial rotation, or internal rotation, moves you toward the midline; lateral rotation, or external rotation, moves you away from the midline.

- *Abduction:* The movement of a limb away from the body.

- *Adduction:* The movement of a limb toward the body.

- *Side Bending:* Bending over to one side; also called lateral flexion.

These primary functional patterns then give way to more refined motions, such as circumduction in a ball-and-socket joint like the shoulder or hip; the elevation and depression that occurs when we shrug our shoulders; pronation and supination in our forearm and foot; dorsiflexion and plantar flexion at the ankle; and inversion and eversion, referring to rotation of the foot around its long axis. These more specific motions are complex and develop out of the primary functional patterns above.

When all six functional motor patterns work together, they create what are often called the primal patterns of gait, squatting, lunging, pulling, pushing, pressing, and twisting. These coordinated movements are what get us from lying on our backs to our bellies, from crawling to creeping to walking and so on. The goal is to use as many of these primal patterns as possible every time we move.

When you need to pick up a glass, your brain doesn't just signal your biceps like calling your best friend on the phone. Movement patterns are orchestrated in the brain's motor system in the frontal lobe. The signal starts with premotor regions for coordinating and planning and ends in the primary motor cortex where the messages are sent down the spinal cord and out to the peripheral nerves to contract muscles and move joints. Repeat a movement enough times and your body hardwires the pattern, so you repeat a movement over and over the same way. That's how a tennis player gets good at serving a ball—practice!

Have you ever seen babies the first time they figure out how to roll over from back to belly? Or the first time they get on all fours? They rock back and forth with glee, like they've just invented something profound. The more parents cheer them on, the more they repeat the movements. Even when we are babies, praise lets us know we are onto something we should repeat. This is what it looks like when primal patterns get hardwired. Starting to collect and organize information and put the data bank together is called neuroplasticity. In other words, the neurons that fire together, wire together.

As the brain's connections get stronger, regions like the cerebellum develop pathways to parts of the brain involved in memory, attention, emotions, and spatial perception. Now movement becomes mostly a memory; you repeat it and become good at it. Interestingly, *the parts of our brain that process movement also process learning and behavior.* Learning is about acquiring knowledge and ability, whereas memory is about retention and storage of knowledge and ability.

Watch infants squat down to pick something up off the floor. They use accurate, clear neural pathways to move *every* joint to squat down, pick up a toy, and return to standing. As we age, however, we use shortcuts to pick up those things—we'll flex only at the hip joint while keeping our knees straight. Alas, mirroring our parents after the age of two seems to override these brilliant and dynamic patterns we once did effortlessly.

Being able to go from crawling to walking depends on how the brain organizes primary patterns and motor programs. Once the cortex of the brain has developed properly and parents have tended to the child appropriately, the child can develop more complex movements, such as running or throwing a ball.

From basic patterns to complex, sequential movements, from birth until about the age of two, we establish a baseline for cognitive choice-making that shapes our physical and emotional behaviors. Gestures become patterns and habits, patterns and habits become movements, and movements become dynamic function.

Think of your reflexes and neurological mechanisms like the letters of the alphabet; you need to create words from those letters. Just like skipping a letter causes words to be misspelled, missing developmental phases or milestones when you are still very young can cause limitations and difficulties in how you perceive, move, feel, and think over your lifetime. Truly, it's a communication breakdown.

Your Brain's Neural Patterns Are Like a Filing Cabinet

An easy way to understand the importance of primal patterns and how they're affected by daily living, repetition, and compensation is with this analogy: You've just gotten a brand-new file cabinet, and you run to the office supply store for color-coded folders and a label maker so everything will be in perfect order. Everything you need to file, like your gas, electric, and water bills, will have their place in their own folder. Utilities are color-coded in red, but each has its own, distinctive folder; home improvements and manuals go in the blue folder. You label everything, excited to remain organized as you fill your file cabinet.

This is what happens between the ages of birth and two, when we develop the basic neural pathways and primal patterns that get us on two feet. Our brains color-code these minute details to then create the folders for each of these dynamic motions. We create a blue one for movements that require flexion, a red one for extension, and so on.

But as babies turn into toddlers and begin to process what they see their parents doing, they start mimicking those movements. The infant who squatted down like a monkey in perfect form to pick up a toy now sees Daddy pick up a book by bending over with his back flat, hips hinged, and straight knees. Suddenly the squatting folder and the lunge folder get mixed together. *Hmm*, goes the toddler's brain. *Daddy picked that book up more quickly than I picked up my toy.* The program for the squat now doesn't look much like a squatting motion at all.

The subfolders in the file cabinet start to get condensed; so, for example gas, electric, and water bills all end up in a single utilities folder. Over time, we even start to mix categories together. So the red utilities folder and blue home improvement folder somehow get filed together—it's like there's now a purple folder. So we have some blue, some red, and some purple folders. Our awesome filing system is slowly falling into disarray.

Although the categories might seem similar, they are in fact different. We do the same thing with movement. Bringing our knee to our chest may be hip flexion, and hinging over at our hip joint to pick up a pencil is hip flexion, too. But they are distinctively different. So suddenly faulty patterns arise—we're bringing the chest to the knee rather than the knee to the chest. Repeat those faulty patterns enough times, and all of the separate folders become one big folder, causing *more* faulty patterns.

The older we get, the more paperwork we have to file. If we don't clean up the file cabinet, it overflows; and sometimes, we just open the file cabinet, put more papers inside, and tell ourselves we'll file them all later. This is how movement patterns get a little funky and ultimately cause unnecessary joint injury.

The pathways that are no longer in use are discarded. Scientifically, this is called synaptic pruning, and it is the brain's way of deleting the neural connections that no longer seem necessary or useful while strengthening the ones we use most often. As we've seen, when we were little, we flexed at the ankles, knees, hip joint, and low back bones to squat down to pick something up off the floor. But as we got older, we developed shortcuts, simply flexing at the hips and reaching down. Though it may have seemed faster and more efficient to flex just one joint, the effect on our low back and knees, and the strain on the muscles on our backside like our hamstrings, paid a dear price. We all but forgot we could squat and move all of those joints—until someone asked us to do it, and we realized that we couldn't anymore!

How our brain decides which connections to prune depends on our life experiences and how recently connections have been used. In much the same way, cells that grow weak from underuse die off through the process of cell death called apoptosis. In general, neuroplasticity is a way for our brain to fine-tune itself for efficiency. It's what makes a baseball player an elite batter just as much as it causes poor motor control and the existence of thought viruses.

The process of neuroplasticity isn't a quick or simple one. Rather, it happens throughout our lifetime and can involve many processes. Along with altering our neural synapses—the structures that permit neurons to pass electrical or chemical signals—neuroplasticity is an intrinsic fundamental neurophysiological component of the constant changes to our bone formation, neurons, vascular tissues, and lymph and glial cells that surround neurons and provide support and insulation both around and between them.

So imagine the widespread issues that can arise if neural pathways are altered. This can inhibit blood flow, excretion, and basic connection to movement, digestion, and function.

The biggest issue, as you clip the good pathways and develop compensations, is that when you bend over, the primary muscles and mechanisms that should be providing stability and ease of movement don't activate properly. Your back suddenly goes into spasms. Your doctor gives you painkillers to mask the agony, but you don't know that the root cause of your pain is not a muscle issue, but the fact that your primal patterns are out of whack. This blurry, gray area of disorganized dysfunction continues, and as soon as you heal, you get injured again. Much like our file cabinet, sometimes we just open the cabinet, pile papers inside, and stop filing altogether. We forget that at one time, we were excited to be organized and in control.

One unfortunate aspect of pain physiology is that the longer pain goes on, the easier it becomes to feel the pain. This is a consequence of a very basic neural process called long-term potentiation, which means that the more times the brain uses a certain neural pathway, the easier it becomes to activate that pathway again. It's like carving a groove through the snow while sledding down a mountain—the more the same path is traveled, the easier it is to fall into that same groove and the faster you get to the bottom of the hill. This is the same process by which we learn habits and develop skills.

Fortunately, as you'll see in Part Two of this book, once a primal pathway of stability has been initiated and reintegrated, you can easily repattern your primal patterns of movement. This is the missing link to restoring efficient, pain-free motion, enhanced performance, and better health.

▶ How We Learn to Compensate— It's All About Repetition

The Beginning of Compensation

When all of our reflexes, reactions, responses, and ultimately our primary movement patterns are available and utilized, physical, emotional, and cognitive growth from childhood to adulthood are wonderfully supported. Far more typical, however, is that many things affect this development and cause lifelong issues that are often treated as symptoms because most doctors don't care enough about ferreting out the cause of our dysfunction. They don't practice prevention—they practice cure, and most have a symptom-based practice.

For instance, your back hurts. A doctor wants you to not feel pain. If they can diagnose your pain or they find something they can fix, fix they will. But just because they find a herniated disc in your back doesn't mean that's the reason your back hurts today. Doctors don't necessarily study neuroplasticity or brain function. Most of them don't realize that motor reflexes and self-protective responses may be disrupted as they develop because of a traumatic event that happened during childhood. These developmental disturbances may then be the underlying cause of adult issues, spanning from our ability to create and maintain healthy attachments to things or people to how we react and respond to loud sounds or current traumatic events. And although psychologists recognize how our past can influence how we learn and perceive our lives today, they don't study neuroplasticity either.

On a larger scale, *life* just gets in the way of resilience and adaptability. Dealing with the enormous stresses of our twenty-first-century society creates roadblocks in our primal pathways and patterns. These roadblocks can cause our body to compensate in how it moves, accelerating body-wide issues from joint pain to neurological or emotional disorders.

Compensation is the way of the body, often to preserve and protect—and you don't know that it's happening. This sets you up for accumulated stress around joints that you need for mobility. What causes this? Our natural tendency to take the path of least resistance—with movement and with so many other issues, both involuntary and voluntary.

The Path of Least Resistance and Involuntary Body Shortcuts

If you live in a suburb and have to drive to get to work in the city every morning, you know that the highway is the fastest way to get downtown—but only if there isn't any traffic. You check your navigation map and see traffic on the highway, so what do you do? You take side streets to get downtown in the same amount of time. You might get to work on time, but you don't take the most direct route. You may have more traffic lights or turns, and you may use more gas, but as long as you get to work on time, you're satisfied with taking the *path of least resistance.* Then, on the weekend when you want to get downtown, when there's no traffic on the highway, by habit, you still take the side streets to get there. After a while, you *always* take the side streets to get downtown; you never take the highway anymore.

Just as you create shortcuts in your daily life to save time and effort, your nervous system is wired to do the same thing. It creates a detour to get around roadblocks—what I call an involuntary body shortcut—just as you take side streets when there's traffic on the highway. The shortcuts your nervous system takes might not be the most direct routes, but they still get you where you want to go. If you don't eliminate your stuck stress, however, over time the side streets become the regular route, sacrificing stability for mobility. Truly, your body becomes exhausted and your gas tank is often empty.

In fact, the detours your nervous system takes create compensatory pathways to execute movements. Your neuronal pathways are like highways. If certain routes on that highway aren't used anymore—like your not using the freeway to get to work because there's too much traffic—your brain puts a detour sign up to say that this road isn't used anymore. The more times your brain takes an involuntary body shortcut—even if it isn't the best and most direct path—the more ingrained the shortcut becomes and the more often your brain uses it to get you to move.

The problem is, when your brain starts to prune the good pathways, over time you're going to have to compensate to move at all. Your brain gets motor amnesia. If you're used to moving in a certain way and then you want to restore a proper stability pathway, your brain is going to be thinking, *Hey, what is this? Can't we just take the shortcut? This is exhausting!*

This might not seem like a big deal, but for sustaining neurological pathways and joint motion efficiency, over time this *becomes* a big deal. Involuntary body shortcuts lead to chronic compensation and misalignments, which decrease performance and efficiency and increase the risk of muscle and joint injuries. Ultimately, this is what keeps an athlete out of the game, and many of us to stop our daily workout routines, by causing unnecessary stress and wear and tear to arise in the vital connective tissues that support and surround our joints.

When a proper pathway is replaced by a shortcut, you still create the movement, but in a less efficient and stable way. For example, if a shortcut is used to raise your arm overhead, your shoulder shrugs before you get there and you probably won't notice the subtle displacement of your shoulder girdle. In fact, if a person uses an involuntary body shortcut when he or she serves during a tennis match, you might not even see it.

Imagine, though, how this affects your tennis serve if you continue to take a shortcut without knowing it. You might hit the ball, but you lose precision and power. Eventually, it will cause shoulder and neck issues, too. Shortcuts lead to chronic compensation and misalignments, less resilience and efficiency, hampered performance, and a higher risk of muscle and joint injuries.

Joints simply don't move well when the motor timing and movement patterns aren't accurate. You can't improve the precision of a tennis swing when neurological stability and control are flawed. Practicing your swing merely makes you a stronger, more dysfunctional athlete who is still neurologically unstable—you get better at managing the shortcut, but in the long term, you'll end up with more problems that perhaps will seem completely unrelated to the power of a swinging arm.

This is what athletes don't know, but it can end their careers before they even get going. In some ways, the remarkable nature of fascia makes athletes more susceptible to injuries, because the demands that they put on their bodies when they move are significantly higher than the demands people make who either work at desk jobs and go to the gym after work or don't exercise at all. It's not so much the skill or ability level that makes a great athlete; it's the ability to stabilize, overcome, and repair issues as they arise so the athlete can continue to perform at a high level.

This is also why so many athletes have short careers. They reach a peak and then sustain an injury that is not given a chance to heal properly. They don't rest enough; they don't do enough recovery; and they don't understand that all the repetitive motions they have done that caused the injury will make things worse unless they take the time to reintegrate and repattern the proper neurological pathways. Most of the athletes I work with have so many layers of compensation that their bodies are like a compensating machine. Yet it only takes a few weeks for them to forge a sturdy foundation of neurological stability—and it will remain sturdy as long as they keep doing their MELT Performance routines. As for the rest of us who aren't elite athletes but possess an inner warrior awaiting its resurrection, even if our repetitive habits are just sitting at a desk all day long, MELT Performance can give our minds and bodies a boost. When we feel resilient, we *want* to move—we get excited to move.

It's time to let your inner warrior emerge and give your inner spirit some attention. You are strong. You are powerful. I want to help you be the best version of yourself and not compromise your life because pain or stress gets in the way. When I say I want to help you improve your performance, I truly mean the resilience of your life.

The cliché about not being able to teach an old dog new tricks *isn't* true. You *can* learn new things—it just takes more mental focus, intention, and specificity to do so. In fact, MELT Performance will show you that you aren't even learning something new; instead, you're restoring what was there long ago and getting back on the right path of stability.

I'll discuss the details of my own story in the next chapter, but for now, it's important to realize although not all pain is the same, it's our brain that always produces our ability to perceive pain. Our sensory system can detect changes in our tissues that alert the brain about problems in the body. This is called nociception. If the brain decodes this information as a threat, you will feel pain but if it's something your brain doesn't sense as a threat, you won't feel pain. In other words, you can have nociception and not feel pain just as much as your brain can send a pain response in the absence of nociception. The simple fact is that pain is both a sensory and an emotional experience.

▌ The Blessing and Curse of Repetition

What makes compensation so entrenched in our body's neurological wiring? There's one very simple explanation: repetition.

Most of us have trained our brains to create and utilize faulty patterns of movement that we have done countless times. What causes this? Daily life—the postures, movements, and emotions that are repeated over the years. As I said in the Introduction, whether we're practicing a golf swing over and over or just sitting at a desk all day, repetition causes stuck stress. The more we repeat a faulty motion or posture, the more the integrity of our connective tissue is challenged. Repetition is truly the blessing and the curse of all movement and function.

The even bigger issue for performance is that stuck stress from repetition affects our neurological stability and control systems. When stability declines, compensation begins.

With stability, timing is everything—but not in the way you might think. Stability occurs without your conscious control, before you even move. But thanks to repetition, your nervous system is already anticipating how you want to move, and off it goes, igniting neurological pathways that stabilize the spine, pelvis, and shoulder girdle.

▌ NeuroStrength Will Rewire Your Pathways

As I said above, muscle strength is not NeuroStrength. As an adult, if you have repeated a movement pattern many times in just one way, you'll find that it's a hard habit to break. Workout know-how will not give you neurological stability unless you undo faulty patterns and replace them with a strong foundation. Fortunately, with NeuroStrength, you can rewire a neuronal pathway in just minutes once you know the right moves.

You'll see how to do this in Part Two. You will learn how to teach your nervous system how to reintegrate the proper timing of motor responses and joint stabilization and then to repattern your movement in a whole new way. Once you know what to do, repetition will no longer be your undoing. Instead, you can train without fear of injury and repeat the movements you need to make in a way what won't slow you down and make you feel like you have to train even harder to progress.

NeuroStrength will cut out the faulty shortcuts and get you back on the neurological stabilization highway. Like the Jedi mind trick in *Star Wars* when Luke Skywalker and Obi-Wan Kenobi are stopped by Stormtroopers. Obi-Wan influences the Stormtrooper's mind and suggests, "These aren't the droids you're looking for." I'm going to show you how to Jedi mind trick your brain, regain mind-body control, and reroute your brain out of its involuntary body shortcuts.

Instead of pruning your good pathways to adapt to the shortcuts of compensating pathways, you're going to undo your old, faulty patterns. I'm going to teach you how to rewire the proper pathways to restore the most efficient, direct routes—no matter what movement you make. This will allow you to improve control, stability, power, speed, and agility—with no downside.

All your movements will become easier and your performance and health stronger. You're going to be protecting your joints for longer. And your brain's going to wake up in a different way.

2

How NeuroStrength Will Improve Your Performance, Eliminate Pain, and Revitalize Your Overall Health

NeuroStrength will rewire your faulty patterns so you can improve how you move, including all aspects of your athletic performance. It will also help you prevent repetitive stress injuries; reduce and prevent pain; improve overall health; regulate stress levels, cellular repair, and digestion; and improve resilience and longevity. It can also have a profound effect on your emotions (as we'll explore in Chapter 3).

▶ Use NeuroStrength to Improve Athletic Performance and Prevent Injuries

As I've said, repetition is the blessing and the curse of athletic performance. Let's say you want to train for a marathon. What is the one thing you know you have to do? Run . . . and run and run yourself right into injury, because the endless repetition causes a degradation in your connective tissue . . . which destabilizes your joints . . . which makes your nervous system compensate . . . which then causes pain . . . which makes your run time decrease . . . which makes you try to push through the pain and keep on going. Until you just can't anymore.

If you're not a professional athlete, getting injured is painful and annoying, but it won't ruin your career. For the pros, injuries cause them to lose momentum, time with the team, and often all of their short-term gains. This makes them feel that they need to train even harder. It also messes with their heads, because they tend to blame themselves, thinking they'll never be able to come back or win again. They know that younger, sturdier, even more competitive athletes are lining up to take their place. If only they knew how MELT Performance could keep them going for decades instead of ending their careers after just a few years and/or one devastating injury.

One of my big gripes about the fitness industry is that people have a preconceived notion that exercise will "fix" what they think is wrong. They tell themselves: *I'm out of shape. I'm overweight. I have back pain. I'll get a membership to a gym and get myself back in shape so I feel better.* So they start to work out, maybe even hiring a trainer for a few sessions to show them the ropes; but if they don't know about NeuroStrength, what they create is a stronger yet more dysfunctional body. They stress out an already stressed-out nervous system to try to acquire control, when all they're really doing is getting better at managing their dysfunction. They get injured and they stop working out and they get out of shape again, and the cycle starts up once more.

There is, in fact, a gamut of physical dysfunction that leads to decreased performance and increased injuries. You've got the person who never engages in any activity on one end, and elite and high-performance athletes on the other. Most people fall somewhere in the middle, especially those like me, who sit at a desk half of the time and exercise or are on the move the other half.

This middle group has the highest tendency for injury, because they believe that after being at their desk all day, going to the gym to work out will erase the negative effects of all that sitting. I wish that were true, but it isn't. As we've seen, your connective tissue is like a sponge, and when you sit for long periods of time, you dry out that sponge. Think back to the spiderweb/cobweb analogy. Your connective tissue's primary purpose is to reserve and store energy so your muscles don't get fatigued and are available for later, adapting itself so that you can function as efficiently as possible for whatever you do the most. It needs to be flexible and adaptable to do its job. If you sit all day, your tissue adapts so you can sit and not stress out your muscles. Over time, it does sitting really well and with great efficiency.

The problem with sitting is that it causes tension on the muscles and fascia that support the spine and compresses the back of your thighs all day. If your back and knees are stiff when you try to return to an upright posture, you're feeling the effects of connective tissue adaptation and dehydration and the loss of fascia's supportive qualities. If fascia loses its resilience and adaptability, your stability and function decline on both a physical and a neurological level. Muscles adapt too, locking short or long, thus becoming inhibited, weak, or delayed when they need to be active. So when you get up to move around, your body's saying: *Hey, wait a minute. I thought you wanted to be good at sitting. Now you want to get up and go to the gym and exercise? I don't know if I'm ready to move you around like that.* Consider this like motor amnesia. Muscles forget that they need to work when you move. You ignore this and go work out anyway, and you feel fine—sort of. Maybe your workout was a little lame and your energy wasn't so great; but you got yourself to the gym, and mentally you feel you've done your body some good.

But then you come home, and what do you do? Sit right back down at the dinner table, and maybe you do some more work at your desk or plop on the sofa and watch TV. When you get up to get ready for bed, you notice your back feels stiff, but you figure that's just a part of working out. No pain, no gain, right? *Wrong.* If you do what many people do and pop a pain reliever or sleep aid before bed, you're actually causing more dysfunction for your nervous system to manage tomorrow. You think the aches and pains you feel are part of an active life—but they are actually distress signals from your body telling you that it needs your help.

It seems to me that one of the worst times to work out is after a full day of sitting, especially if you're running late and skip your warmup—and then you get injured. But it wasn't just skipping the warmup that caused the injury. It was the rushing, the expectations driving you, and, most of all, the accumulated stress in your neurofascial system that you didn't realize needed to be addressed. Simply put, your body wasn't prepared to execute what you wanted, but you did it anyway.

It's hard to get started when you don't know that your connective tissue is losing its resilience. This is precisely what makes the nervous system compensate in all the wrong ways. It's a neurological imbalance that occurs very quickly. Luckily, MELT gives you the ability to take care of this and was designed to restore the resilience of your fascial system and improve neurological efficiency. It's the best pre-workout system you can have. Hydrated fascia creates a supportive environment like flexible scaffolding, allowing muscles to connect and bones to float so the spaces between them, your joints, remain stable. This allows every cell, nerve, muscle, and organ architectural support to function more efficiently. With MELT Performance, you divert your brain's attention from what's moving to what's staying stable. Then, you reintegrate and repattern new pathways back to their ideal state to improve joint alignment, enhance muscle timing, and prevent injuries from happening.

As you'll see in Part Two, once you start doing the MELT Performance sequences, you'll immediately feel the changes in your alignment and posture, and you'll start feeling stronger. When you first begin, you'll do MELT Performance about three times a week, for only ten to fifteen minutes a day. After a while, you can hit these routines just on recovery or training days to decrease any tendency to get injured. Start by doing one hip stabilization technique, and then go out on your run. If you're a competitive athlete, it's better to do MELT Performance routines on training days rather than performance days, when you're focused on competition and coming out on top rather than on movement and stability. One of the most important aspects of restoring sensorimotor control is engagement in the process. While this may seem like common sense, many injured athletes don't respect a simple truth: Every movement is a skill. To acquire a skill, focus and repetition are required.

▶ Pain Is Both a Sensory and an Emotional Experience

As a competitive athlete, I've broken bones (seven out of ten toes!), sprained ankles, suffered contusions, and felt impact assaults on my body from playing contact sports. I've had bike accidents, tumbled down stairs, had concussions and car accidents . . . you name it. Most of us have suffered painful accidents, illness, sports injuries, or stress injuries, and all of us have the normal issues from daily living causing pain that can quickly take over our lives.

Pain isn't a topic most of us want to discuss. In fact, most of us either ignore it or wait to talk about it with our doctors—which is a shame, as we should all be *proactive* about our health. But instead, we are mostly *reactive* to pain; that is, we deal with it only when we are enduring it. In my two decades of obsessing over the topic of pain and how to eliminate it, I've recognized that the true problem with pain is our lack of understanding the pain signal to begin with.

Pain is a vital function of our neurological system—an internal alarm to notify us of a potential or actual problem, injury, or issue. The complexities of pain are far-reaching, as they span both sensory and emotional experiences, both past and present, and they are easily recalled from our memories, beliefs, fears, or anxieties about pain.

Aside from witnessing pain with thousands of clients over the years, I know about it from difficult personal experiences.

I'll discuss the details of my own story in the next chapter, but for now, it's important to realize that pain is both a sensory and an emotional experience. Past loss and emotional trauma can play an important role in how we perceive pain and relate to it. Fear and anxiety also play a significant role in pain sense and transmission. The process is complex, and it's modulated by our responses, facilitation, and inhibitory interactions that aren't controlled by our conscious thought. I had a client, for instance, who came to see me about pain in his shoulder, but the pain was actually due to an irritation of his diaphragm that followed gallbladder surgery. What's compelling is that this patient's shoulder pain came on more than a *year* after that surgery, so it wasn't even considered as a side effect of a known trauma to his body.

When it comes to experiencing pain, you aren't alone. Millions upon millions of people suffer with persistent pain caused by a vast array of issues. But the way pain is usually treated is disheartening. People go to a doctor, and when the doctor tells them that the medication being prescribed takes weeks to work, let alone that they may be on that medication for years and have a number of possible side effects they nod, say *Okay*, and are still in pain while they wait for the pain-killing effects to kick in. Most of these people aren't aware that they can go to a hands-on therapist for pain relief or take classes that will allow their bodies to go through a much more natural healing process with long-term results and no negative side effects. Or they aren't willing to do that. We're as much victims of our current medical establishment as the medical practitioners themselves. And we are all waiting for a quick-fix remedy. Many people believe that a therapist should instantaneously "fix" the problem in one session, and if they don't feel any better after an hour, forget it. I'll say it again, self-care is your best health care system.

I saw this play out every time I worked with a group of athletes. When I asked them how many had chronic pain, no one ever raised a hand. But if I asked, "So none of you has ever injured yourself or had a joint or muscle issue you feel holds you back from achieving peak performance?" Then every hand went up, and I got a wide range of specifics. So I realized I had to redefine pain or ask the question in a way that created rapport with and understanding in the athletes. You might want to say "aches" or "stiffness" rather than "pain." But whatever you call it, stuck stress in your connective tissue is part of the issue making you feel those things.

Part of the problem with discussing pain is that there are many types and varying degrees of pain within two traditional categories: acute pain and chronic pain. *Acute pain* is traditionally considered a pain caused by a traumatic event or accident. You get hit by a car, fall down a flight of stairs, trip on the sidewalk, bang your head on a cabinet door, or cut your finger when you're slicing tomatoes. You know exactly what happened to cause the pain. When you have an acute trauma, pain and inflammation are a good thing, and they're both part of the healing process. Pain is your brain's way of drawing your attention to a stimulus it sees as a potential threat to your well-being.

Chronic pain is traditionally believed to be caused by genetic or long-term disease conditions such as diabetes, osteoarthritis, or asthma or by traumatic injuries that permanently damage tissues. These conditions cause low-grade inflammation, a side effect of the disease, rather than of the healing process. Sometimes, however, chronic pain comes from nothing specific, in the absence of any tissue damage, and is often elusive and resistant to medication and therapy.

Pain caused by a traumatic event is a measure that your body uses to prevent you from moving so the injury doesn't get worse, but chronic pain is very rarely preventative. It's actually a side effect of another problem. You have diabetes; this causes neuropathy (nerve numbness or weakness), which leads to leg pain. The illness of diabetes does not itself cause leg pain, neuropathy does.

There is also a subcategory of chronic pain that I call *sudden chronic pain*. This is a pain that comes on suddenly but is not caused by a specific trauma, although it can cause as much discomfort as acute pain. You bend over to pick up a pencil, and your back goes out and you can't move. Bending over to pick up a pencil is not a traumatic event. Instead, accumulated stress led to sudden chronic pain.

Acute pain is a normal sensation triggered in the nervous system to alert you to possible injury and the need to take care of yourself; chronic pain is different. Chronic pain persists. Pain signals keep firing in the nervous system for weeks, months, even years. There may have been an initial trauma—surgery, serious infection—or there may be an ongoing cause of pain—arthritis, cancer—but some people suffer chronic pain in the absence of any past injury or evidence of body damage. Many chronic pain conditions affect older adults. Common chronic pain complaints include headache, low back pain, muscle pain, joint pain, and neurogenic pain (pain resulting from damage to the peripheral nerves or to the central nervous system itself), and psychogenic pain (pain not due to past disease or injury or any visible sign of damage inside or outside the nervous system). It can cause our neuroelectrochemical systems to go haywire, creating an inflammatory response that works against our natural healing processes.

Chronic pain often results when there are pre-pain signals, such as constant achiness or stiffness in one or more joints, muscle fatigue, or soreness that goes on days and days after a workout. This can then lead to other, more noticeable symptoms like a buzzy kind of tingle down your arm or little twinges in your back when you first get out of bed in the morning. However, these types of issues seem to dissipate once you start moving or you get used to it and stop thinking about it. Basically, we ignore pre-pain signals because we think they're normal. Athletes, in particular, train themselves to become desensitized to pain. They learn to tune it out, push it out, and not let it stop them—until it gets really bad. Usually by that time, the damage is severe—and so are the repercussions.

The Brain Pain Game

When you're in pain, you've got to acknowledge it and try to get to the root of its source. Have you ever seen a football player get clobbered after a much-needed touchdown? All of his teammates pile on top of him. I would think, *Doesn't that hurt?* Most likely, no, because football players are so used to getting clobbered, and the adrenaline pumping through their bodies desensitizes them in the moment. The touchdown-scorer gets up afterward, shakes it off, and goes right back to the game. He didn't feel a thing. That's because pain in and of itself is a brain thing. It's the brain pain game. Your brain figures out that if the pain is not going to save you or protect you—such as a surfer getting bitten by a shark and then swimming back to shore without even a twinge of pain until she knows she's safe—the adrenaline is going to kick in and push the pain away. If that surfer had been in agony, she would have drowned, so her brain shuts off the pain response until it knows the body is out of immediate danger.

In other words, if the pain response is going to hinder your immediate well-being, you probably won't feel it.

When I was getting my master's degree in anatomy, I was taught that the majority of proprioceptive cells, which receive stimuli from within the body and respond to joint position and movement, were in the muscles. That was incorrect. It turns out that there are *ten times more* sensory nerve endings in *fascia* than in muscle. We need to realize this because the information from proprioceptors comes through the sensory nerve endings. Superficial fascia, the layer that adheres on the underside of your skin is the environment that billions of sensory nerve endings live in, so the health of this tissue is critical.

This is where MELT Performance is such a game-changer. Through the MELT Performance moves and sequences, not only will you give your fascia the care it needs, but you will reprogram the faulty neurological patterns caused by normal, daily repetitions that initiated the problems in the first place.

Even better, the new patterns take effect immediately. One of the reasons I love to work with athletes is that they do their MELT Performance routines faithfully. I follow up with them, they ask questions, and if they're having trouble with a certain move, I work with them to fix it. Two weeks later, they're raring to go because the pain is gone; but I tell them to wait, because now that we've gotten pain levels down, it's time to restore optimal functioning, movement patterns, and joint stability. It'll take only another week. Once I get them there, I can then give them a whole new process, which allows them to get back to doing the repetition they need to do for their sport. Creating better stability pathways before they go back to repetition gives the body more precision.

One of the most gratifying aspects of my work is seeing how well and how quickly this process works. It takes so little time and energy to undo years, if not decades, of damage. People get on the roller in pain, and they get off it with that wow-it's-amazing-how-much-better-I-feel-already look on their faces. I tell them to keep doing exactly what they learned. That's what transforms them—they feel MELT working. Movement starts in the mind, and intention creates action.

▶ Use NeuroStrength to Improve Your Overall Health

Your brain is very clever. It's always looking for the path of least resistance. To do what it needs to do, it's designed to figure out easy ways around the roadblock, to create a detour and it's extremely good at doing that.

If your nervous system is exhausted, in fact, it doesn't try to pep you up. Instead, it slows down your metabolism and shunts energy away from anything that's not vital—such as the quantity of hair on your head, the amount of fluid in your eyes, or the strength of your nails—as these aren't life-threatening issues like heart rate and adequate respiration. This is how the nervous system reserves energy for important processes. But when your metabolism slows down, waste accumulates, nutrient absorption declines, and you're accelerating not only your tendency toward pain, but the aging process as well. You have a greater tendency to develop an autoimmune issue, malnutrition, cell dehydration, and all sorts of other health issues.

This is one of the reasons why people often get sick after they've been very stressed. Stress can come from a huge project at work, your needing to take care of a sick family member, or a 5K race that you've been training for. When you pushed yourself out of your comfort zone, your immune system reacted to tell you that you needed to rest and recuperate. You know why? Because immune function originates in your connective tissue. If the normal cell processes in your connective tissue can't occur because that tissue is dehydrated, your nervous system starts pumping out pro-inflammatory hormones in response, and so you feel awful.

This phenomenon is incredibly common, but if you go to a doctor, chances are pretty good he or she won't explain it to you and instead will just tell you, "Oh, you're stressed out. Take it easy and you'll be fine."

By addressing the proper functioning of your connective tissue, reintegrating and repatterning movement, and decreasing compensation, MELT Performance will strengthen your neurological regulators of stress, repair, and digestion, not to mention your immune system. It is an incredibly effective way to help your body function optimally.

▶ Use NeuroStrength to Help Regulate Your Stress Levels, Cellular Repair, and Digestion

Everything from thinking to breathing to digestion is linked to our nervous system. It controls how we receive, use, and react to information every minute of every day. The science behind most fitness concepts is rooted in muscle anatomy and physiology, with the primary focus on the musculoskeletal system. But the nervous system must be a key component of this mix if we want to improve the body's stability, function, and movement. Without it, joint compression, misalignment, and pain are inevitable side effects of exercise. So if we can identify the forces that occur in our bodies during exercise, we can understand the cause of these consequences and take steps to eliminate them. Exercise and activity are good for the body, so the models and methods need to evolve. Incorporating the nervous system is the starting point.

How Joe Got Out of Pain

Before he came to me for help, Joe had back pain and right knee pain caused by, he was certain, very tight hamstrings. He had fixated on the notion that he needed to stretch his hamstrings, mostly his right leg, because a yoga instructor and his general practitioner had told him they were very tight. Joe was an avid cyclist, both indoor and on the road, so this seemed obvious to him as he realized he never spent much time stretching after strenuous rides. So he started doing yoga. After doing the same Downward Dog pose that he'd been doing twice a week, every week, for six months, he felt a "strain-like burn with a sound like a tiny pop" in his right buttock. His doctor told him that he had strained his sacrotuberous ligaments and hamstring tendons—the supportive connective tissue attaching the hamstring muscle to the sits bone—and sent him to a physical therapist, who gave him rehab exercises. After a few months Joe's leg felt better, and he went back to his twice-weekly yoga sessions.

One year later, Joe got hurt again. His right knee ached, his low back pain returned, his hamstrings were still tight, but this time his left leg was injured.

Luckily, Joe found his way to my indoor cycling class. In a conversation about his seat position, I mentioned that his backside looked compromised. "Funny enough," he said, "my hamstrings and back are totally out of whack. You can see it?" I told him to look at the MELT website because MELTing is what he really needed—not stretching. The next week he came back to my class begging for a private session.

We quickly discovered that the source of his issue was not his hamstrings—it was his *pelvis.* His hamstrings became adaptively shortened, trying desperately to keep his sacroiliac joint from shearing. The SI joint is the oddly shaped joint where our pelvic bones, called the ilia, connect to our sacrum. The sacrum looks like a bridge keystone, snuggly contained in its place through ligaments and essentially the force and integrity of our fascial system. His SI joint was compromised. Due to the brain's inability to "fix" the situation, it adapted. It protected the joint by inhibiting sensorimotor response. This adaptive shortening caused other muscles to become inhibited, limiting his range of movement. His neurological system was basically telling his hamstrings to help keep his SI joint stable. By not knowing what was actually causing the problem, he had treated only the symptom of tight hamstrings. This reduced the protective response and increased his potential for injury. His hamstrings might have stopped hurting in the short term, but the instability and imbalances that had caused him to strain his hamstrings in the first place hadn't been fixed. That's why his pain had returned and even gotten worse.

Joe and I set out to create a MELT Map to address his real issues. Once we resolved the problem in his connective tissue, we focused on reintegrating his pelvic stability and sensorimotor control with MELT Performance. This allowed him to regain stability in his joints and to better align his form, which took the strain and pull out of his hamstrings and alleviated his low back ache. This was when magic really happened. We discovered that an old injury from a fall on his skateboard twenty years before was still causing issues, and I was able to help him restore the proper timing and function of his hip stabilizers. His knees stopped hurting for the first time in twelve years.

Joe had only four sessions with me, and it took six weeks of focused work for him to get out of pain. *Only six weeks to undo twelve years of pain*, and for the first time in his life he could bend over and touch the floor without straining!

Joe was able to sustain the changes we made and successfully reinforce the newly reintegrated neurological pathway and proper firing pattern in his sensorimotor system. As his body maintained the right changes, he was able to use the MELT Performance techniques less often. But he continued to MELT daily, most often spending fifteen or twenty minutes while watching the news when he got home from work.

Two years later, Joe not only practices yoga with joy, he has run two half-marathons and one full marathon and is now training for his first triathlon. Joe, by the way, is fifty-six years old! And he's never felt better.

Essential Elements of the Nervous System

The three elements of healthy living are

- the health of the nervous system,

- the body's ability to produce, utilize, and maintain a chemical and hormonal balance, including metabolism, and

- the quality and integrity of the connective tissue.

The aspects of the nervous system that we are the most concerned about in relation to living an active, healthy, pain-free life are all housed within the autonomic nervous system (ANS). Its functions are massive, outside of our conscious control, and critical to every moment of every day. These functions are

- Responsiveness to movement and changes in our external environment

- Regulation of stress, cellular repair, and digestion

- Repair of all systems of the body through activation of our powerful, innate healing mechanisms

- GPS-like monitoring of the body's center of gravity to allow us to move with minimal compression of joints and organs

How the Nervous System Works

"Why am I always so exhausted?" Patty asked me. "I exercise every day, I try not to overeat; I mean, I'm doing all the right things, so why is my body failing me? I train harder and barely eat but gain more weight. I'm constipated, bloated, my joints ache, and I can't even think straight anymore. I even recently left my kids in the driveway after I got in the car and started driving down our street. Something's really wrong with me. Maybe I have early-onset dementia."

This is a perfect example of a thought virus, which I'll discuss in Chapter 3. I asked Patty to elaborate on her life and out came a common story. She lives in New York City. She has three kids and a full-time job, her husband travels a lot for work, they frequently spend over their budget, and she's left juggling their kids' activities in between her workday priorities. Patty does what most of us do. We take care of everything around us except ourselves. The stress we bring in outweighs our body's natural ability to repair and restore so we can start off tomorrow in a balanced state. So why is Patty so exhausted? Is her body failing her? Or is she failing to take action in response to the messages her nervous system is sending her?

The nervous system is complex, so explaining how it functions is complicated. Even neuroscientists can't explain every aspect of the nervous system. But much like anatomy, to understand the system's parts and functions, science does what it does with all systems: It cuts the system up into subparts to try to define it and learn how it works.

On a scientific level, the nervous system is basically composed of two main parts: the central nervous system, or CNS (the brain and spinal cord), and the peripheral nervous system, or PNS (the peripheral nerves). Our brain acts like an antenna for our body, as opposed to a one-way command base. This antenna relies on information and communication from the body in order to generate accurate responses. The CNS and PNS work together to manage incoming information as well as manage what's going on inside our body without our voluntary or conscious intervention.

Housed within the PNS are two other subsets that monitor our external and internal environments and send information back to the brain for processing and taking action. The sensory-somatic nervous system (SSNS) monitors our external environment and regulates our common senses, such as touch, taste, smell, hearing, and sight, enabling us to respond to our surroundings. Our ability to create movement and react to changes in our external environment relies on the accuracy of sensory response. In order for a suitable motor response to occur, the brain must receive accurate, timely information from our common senses.

The autonomic nervous system (ANS) monitors our body's internal environment. It is a self-managing system that is always working, mostly without our conscious control. The ANS regulates the functions of the internal organs and the glands to maintain homeostasis, or internal balance. It also regulates all vital functions, such as heart rate, digestion, salivation, breathing, perspiration, and pupil diameter.

When it comes to how we autonomically process and manage incoming stress from our external environment as well as sustain balance and control of our internal environment, we need to cut the nervous system up yet again—into three exquisite regulators of stress, repair, and digestion called the sympathetic, parasympathetic, and enteric nervous systems.

The Sympathetic and Parasympathetic Nervous Systems

The sympathetic and parasympathetic nervous systems operate together like a seesaw to help the body negotiate stress and maintain internal balance by elevating and reducing the body's vital functions. Think of the sympathetic nervous system as the body's *stress regulator* and the parasympathetic nervous system as the body's *restore regulator.* The stress regulator increases heart rate, perspiration, and pupil dilation in response to what it perceives as incoming, external stress. The restore regulator relaxes these same functions to restore the body's internal balance. Our ability to respond to stress and return to balance directly correlates to how healthy we are.

A broad range of circumstances can end up triggering the stress regulator. In fact, it responds to anything that it perceives as stress, such as watching television, multitasking, reading, exercising, walking up stairs, gardening, crossing the street, and working. Although each of these activities requires varying responses from the stress regulator, they all involve brain communication—seeking commands for how to react, adjust the internal systems, and, when necessary, keep the body safe.

With each stressful moment, ideally the restore regulator kicks into action to bring down the stress responses over the course of the day. However, in many people's lives, modern technology has led to a busier lifestyle. People work more hours and expend more energy to manage their modern lives. Our brain can't process that much stress every single day without rest and repair. The stress regulator is in a constant state of management, so restore and repair occurs mostly when we're asleep. And here's the problem: When you ask people whether they fall asleep easily and stay asleep for eight hours and wake up feeling rested, most answer "No." The incoming stress outweighs the time we spend in the restore and repair mode. This tilts the seesaw so much that the restore regulator is unable to bring about internal balance— even at night when it's ideally dominant and when most cellular repair is supposed to occur. If you don't get a restful night's sleep, you wake up the next morning with a backlog of stress in your body. Only when the restore regulator is functioning efficiently can intuition, healing, cell renewal, and rapid eye-movement (REM) sleep, among other functions, occur.

If the body's self-healing mechanism is unable to activate, multiple systemic problems are created. When the stress regulator is dominating the seesaw, the energy required for basic day-to-day functioning becomes depleted. The autonomic monitor slows or even shuts down any daily processes that aren't necessary to keep us alive. Fluid in the eyes, salivation in the mouth, and hydration needed for digestion decrease, and metabolism and circulation decline. Eventually, more systemic problems—such as increased toxicity, inflammation, acidity, and poor nutrient absorption—will arise.

As the stress and repair regulators fall out of balance, more symptoms arise, and we don't realize it's an effect of something far greater. We gain weight, we feel exhausted, we can't digest food properly, and we are constipated, grumpy, and anxious.

The Enteric Nervous System

When the stress and restore regulators are functioning inefficiently, multiple problems ensue for the third, and what I'd consider the most critical, component of the ANS: the enteric nervous system. This is the *gut regulator*, which directly manages every aspect of your intestines—digestion, absorption, and transportation of nutrients.

Digestion is a mechanical, chemical, and absorptive process that starts in the mouth and ends at the excretory tract, with many organs participating in between. This highly intricate system has more parts than the transmission of a car. Neurotransmitters produced in the gut regulate the gut-brain relationship.

The gut is as powerful as it is complex, yet the field of neurogastroenterology is a relatively new area of research. In 1996, Dr. Michael Gershon at Columbia University coined the term *second brain* to describe the gut. There are more than one million nerve cells in the small intestine, which is the same number of nerve cells in the spinal cord. If we add the nerve cells of the esophagus, stomach, and large intestine, the gut has more nerve cells than the entire rest of the body.

The gut regulator is designed to operate for the most part independently of the brain and functions most efficiently when it is autonomous. In fact, what we eat and how the enteric nervous system breaks down and transports nutrients to the brain are key factors in our overall brain health. We now know that sugar is like heroin in the body and can alter the function of the pleasure centers of the brain. When our stress and restore regulators are unable to maintain internal balance, the gut regulator becomes distressed. Poor diet, allergies, environmental toxins, UV rays, nicotine, caffeine, alcohol, and pharmaceuticals, not to mention the stress of everyday living, wreak havoc on the gut regulator, which in turn leads to even more stress/restore imbalance, which further causes the gut-brain disconnect. When this happens, various organs of the gut independently plead for attention and inundate the brain with multiple mixed messages.

In the brain's attempt to neurologically respond to all of these incoming messages, more chemical chaos and distress is created for the gut to manage. It sends signals in the form of subtle symptoms, such as indigestion, constipation, backache, headache, acid reflux, cramps, and even depression. This is the body's warning system. These symptoms all indicate the presence of inflammation—the aging accelerator known as the silent killer. All of these signals alert us that something's not right, yet most of us just pop a pill to ease the symptoms or ignore them until they get more persistent.

When we ignore or suppress these signals, the gut gets more disrupted, and the inflammation cycle escalates into other, more serious problems. Gut imbalances become chronic, digestive and immune disorders arise, and toxicity skyrockets. The mixed messages become error messages, and the gut neurologically short-circuits.

When the body becomes overloaded with inflammation, the brain gets too many messages, and in some ways, it causes a gut-brain disconnect, shutting down communication in order to support, protect, and stabilize the other organs. Joints become chronically inflamed. Energy transfer becomes impaired, and foggy brain, improper muscle contraction and firing, chronic symptoms, pain, and fatigue quickly follow. Chronic inflammatory issues arise, such as sinusitis, arthritis, tonsillitis, dermatitis, colitis, and a long list of other disorders that end in -itis.

You now feel exhausted, you can't sleep, you can't eat certain foods, your skin becomes lackluster, and you start gaining excess weight. You become like Patty—exhausted, bloated, and distracted.

So, what can you do to keep the restore regulator functioning efficiently? Eliminating or reducing the intake of stressors is a good first step, but as many of my clients point out, they can't give away their kids, quit their job, and move to a resort and live there for free. Real life is a real bitch. It exists whether we like it or not. However, we can in fact stop this dysfunctional cascade. In order to boost the restore regulator and maintain the internal balance of the ANS, you must first appreciate the communication that occurs beyond the brain.

Keeping Up with the Joneses

This is a lot of information for anyone to absorb, I know. So to simplify the story I'll share my family analogy. Think of your nervous system as a high-society power couple—let's call them the Jones family. Charlie and Pat Jones are a very well-known, influential couple with fraternal twins, Sam and Pam, and a brilliant younger sibling, Ernie.

Charlie and Pat are the equivalent of your central nervous system (your brain and spinal cord) and your peripheral nervous system (your body and nerves). Charlie is a busy executive of a multibillion-dollar company and is always working. He doesn't have time to monitor or regulate the day-to-day events in his home. Pat is a socialite who is more concerned about what the world is saying about her family than in paying attention to the children. Yes, she spends more time than Charlie overseeing the home, but she must carefully manage how her family interacts with and is perceived by the outside world. Pat doesn't take care of the household on her own, because she is a very busy woman. She has a personal assistant and a nanny.

Sally, the personal assistant, is like your sensory-somatic nervous system, regulating your five common senses. She is in charge of monitoring the external environment of the household and any incoming information and gossip about the family. Annie, the nanny, is the equivalent of your autonomic nervous system. She looks after the three children, Sam, Pam, and Ernie, and is in charge of monitoring the day-to-day goings-on inside the home and making sure the kids are okay.

Like many families, the children are truly the ones who run the household. When the kids are in their routine and content, the household runs smoothly. The two twins—like your sympathetic and parasympathetic nervous systems—are particularly active. Sam is the high-energy, ADD kid. He's the one with his fingers all over everything—playing with Xbox and his action heroes, playing a board game, and talking on the phone with a friend, all at the same time and while making a mess throughout the house. Sam is like the sympathetic nervous system, the stress regulator—always on, always going.

Pam is the polar opposite of Sam, despite being his twin. She's the Om Shanti child. She likes organization. She likes detail. Everything's pink in her room. Her bed is always made, and she likes using the vacuum cleaner. Because Pam loves to be organized, during the day she tries to clean up after her brother. Sam usually protests because he's not done using his toys, so most of the time, she waits until Sam is asleep to clean up the mess. Pam is like the parasympathetic nervous system, the restore and repair regulator—working when you sleep.

Ernie, the third child, is a genius. He is the equivalent of your enteric nervous system—smart and independent, but sensitive too. He started reading books when he was two years old, does the family taxes, likes to read about quantum physics, is designing an addition to the family garage, and is currently writing a dissertation on some abstract concept no one has ever thought of before. Ernie is a multitasker, and his parents are clever enough to realize that they should just let him do his own thing. There are even times when Ernie's parents go to him for advice and assistance. He operates best when he is left alone to give each project his full focus. He is happiest when his siblings are content, the household runs smoothly and efficiently, and he is not distracted by hyperactivity or unrest.

When Pam comes out at night to clean up and makes too much noise, she wakes up her brother Sam, so she goes back to her room and in the morning the mess still exists. When Pam can't clean up, you feel exhausted in the morning and sluggish all day. You grab coffee to wake yourself up—which just further high-wires Sam. You aren't helping.

Now, Pam not being able to clean up the house occasionally isn't a big deal, but if Sam goes into Pam's room and starts messing around with her things, you'll get a more noticeable response. Pam tells Annie, the nanny, that Sam is not playing nice. In your body, you get more symptoms. You're not only exhausted, you're constipated, you're grabbing anything to eat in the afternoon—a doughnut, cookies, or fast food—hoping for an energy boost. This causes a bigger disruption because now Ernie's being bothered too.

If Sam gets into Ernie's room, this causes far greater body responses. Because remember, Sam is smart. He doesn't bother to alert Annie; he goes right to Pat and expresses his frustration. That's you waking up in the middle of the night because you have to pee and then being unable to fall back asleep again. In the morning you wake up exhausted, and now you seem to be having trouble digesting food. You have more heartburn and constipation. You feel bloated, irritated, depressed, or anxious.

If you do what most people do and just expect things to go back to normal, Ernie gets annoyed. He doesn't even bother to tell Annie or Pat, he starts calling Charlie directly, who's in China working on the biggest deal of his career.

Now this is the critical part of the story. Charlie needs to take Ernie seriously. If he says to Ernie, "Hey, I'm busy, that's why we have a nanny, go tell her, I don't have time for this, figure this out yourself, you're the smartest one in the family," etc., well, now you've got a real problem.

But if you think about it, this is often how we react when our body isn't performing the way we want it to. Like Charlie ignoring Ernie's concerns, we ignore the signs of distress and just pop a pill so we don't feel pain or take a laxative or other products to eliminate the symptom.

The Moral of the Story: Don't be Charlie! Children can't manage or run a household. If you aren't home as a parent to sustain balance, it's just a matter of time before you come home to charges of tax evasion, divorce papers, and your house burned down. In this instance, don't be like the Joneses.

Let's take this analogy back to the reality of a human body—specifically, yours. When all aspects of your nervous system operate in an efficient, balanced way, so too do your body's systems. Your body looks and feels great. Your energy is vibrant. Your health is optimal. When you actively maintain balance and Autopilot efficiency—in other words, you continuously and consciously look out for your long-term wellness—your body's efficient, optimal state will be sustained.

If, instead, you stop eating well, grab food on the run, skip exercise, drink coffee to stay awake, and forget about drinking water, your body will begin to lose its ability to restore and repair itself. Over time, you may begin gaining weight. You might become restless or develop achiness in your back and neck. You might suddenly have difficulty falling or staying asleep. You might try to ignore these kinds of things, but if your daily habits don't improve, new and more acute symptoms will eventually arise, such as headaches or indigestion, constipation, or diarrhea after eating. These kinds of symptoms are subtle signs of nervous system distress.

Acute symptoms are the equivalent of your gut regulator (Ernie) sending mayday signals to try to get the attention of your brain (Charlie). These signs of gut imbalance are not the only symptoms that need attention, either. They're also cries that the body's regulating system needs attention, too!

As the unpleasant symptoms inevitably persist, you will eventually search for some relief. You'll pop an antacid, go on a crash diet, or maybe take a laxative—any of which will only compound your problems and add to the stress already in your body. Now you are masking and suppressing your body's distress signals, only to find the symptoms escalating and turning into new problems.

At this point, Annie, the nanny, goes into "safety mode," just like your computer when it's low on memory. It may still operate, but your programs don't work properly and some may not work at all, like chronic issues: migraines, irritable bowel syndrome (IBS), depression, chronic fatigue, or disease (dis-ease). Living stops being easy.

You may be thinking, "I already have a bunch of those symptoms! Now what?" The good news is that it's not too late. You need to learn how to access the regulators *directly*. To do this, you need to MELT—that is, quiet the stress regulator and focus on helping the restore regulator to come back online so that your gut regulator can get back to work.

This is the first step in getting your "family" back in balance!

Many times, I have heard in my practice, "Why did my body fail me?" In reality, our bodies don't fail us. We fail to stay *connected to* our bodies and to *listen to* them. You can't will your body to stay well. You must learn to check in and stay tuned in to your internal environment so when you aren't thinking about what's going on in your body, it functions efficiently without your conscious intervention.

You are the responsible adult. You are the parent. You need to go in and cultivate the relationship with your nervous system—your own CNS and PNS power couple—so that everything it controls works better. You need to take care of your children and not always rely on the nanny to keep everything working well.

But we're not taught to do that. We're taught to ignore pain and distress or take a pill. When I ask my clients how many medications they take, most of them take at least three (usually for depression, high cholesterol, and high blood pressure), sometimes with two more to treat side effects of the first three!

If you don't check in to your body, care for yourself, nurture yourself, and do what you need to do to help yourself stay balanced, it's just a matter of time before the kids run the show. It's time to listen to your body and take control, to not judge what you've done in the past but move forward with confidence about your well-being.

▶ Use NeuroStrength to Improve Your Longevity and Resilience

Most people don't think about aging until it starts to happen—and then, of course, all we want to do is reverse it. Instead, imagine how good it would be to prevent issues associated with aging in the first place.

Can you catch cell dehydration before it causes you problems? Yes, you can. Adenosine triphosphate (ATP) is the organic compound that transports chemical energy within cells for metabolism and is considered "molecular currency" for our bodies. As we age, our ability to transfer energy and use this currency declines. Research suggests that neurological alteration in the aging brain is caused in part by a decline in cellular energy metabolism, and the most cutting-edge research is looking at issues such as cellular hydration and the use of discrete stabilizing mechanisms within our body's cellular structures as a way to decrease cellular energy loss. This means that NeuroStrength and the hydration techniques of MELT could be the doorway to keeping ATP in production as we age, which would increase longevity.

In addition, the most common tactic for age reversal is to stay active. But as you get older, you get more sedentary, you move cautiously, meaning you're having to think about moving. Your body can only compensate so much. It's like your computer always being on safety mode—it still functions, but very slowly and inefficiently. In fact, walking around more cautiously can actually cause more problems. The more you *think* about walking, the more you interrupt the involuntary mechanisms of stability. You shouldn't have to think about walking when you walk. When you find yourself looking down at the ground as you walk, your brain is telling you it needs to see what it's walking on to get you where you want to go. Your head being down stops you from seeing what's in front of you and keeping your stability reflexes and mechanisms functioning properly. This allows compensation to kick in.

Just as many people do a short stretching routine as a warmup to their regular exercise routine, I want you to think of MELT Performance as its own unique kind of warmup. Not one that will literally "warm up" your muscles, but one that can prepare you for both physical and emotional well-being.

I also want you to rethink what fitness is. It's not just about having strong muscles and sturdy bones and flexibility and a well-oiled cardiovascular system. It's about *resilience*. This resilience is ultimately what will create the longevity everybody craves. MELT Performance is really all about having a *resilient* body, not just a *fit* body.

What ages people or makes them feel old is the inability to efficiently adapt and change. As I've said before, forget that old cliché about not being able to teach an old dog new tricks. Old dogs can learn new tricks all the time, if they're motivated enough (especially when your rewards are extra-tasty!). Older people can, too, especially when they aren't hampered by self-defeating or limited options.

For instance, if your knees are hurting you because you don't exercise and you need to lose some weight, and you're going to visit a friend who lives on the third floor of an apartment building, your first thought is probably going to be, "I sure hope there's an elevator because I'm really not in the mood for climbing any stairs." Your options are limited, and feeling your limitations and anticipating a problem are exhausting, which compounds the problem of what inactivity does to a body. You're not living in the present moment anymore; you're living in the hypothetical future, and if it looks grim, heck, you might not see your friend again if it means walking up those stairs to do so.

NeuroStrength is about having the resilience to adapt, respond, and repeat. It allows you to quickly adapt to any physical situation. You can climb up those three flights of stairs without even thinking about it!

So although there's no shortcut, there is a simple way to improve your longevity and resilience. You will have to invest some time and effort into learning what to do to make these changes, but once you master the MELT Performance routines, you'll spend just a few minutes a day doing them—and the rest of your life reaping the rewards.

3

NeuroStrength and Your Emotions

Dealing with Instability on a Soul Level

In the aftermath of 9/11, my understanding of stress injuries took on new meaning. For more than a decade, I'd been working on athletes who had been injured and had experienced pain. I had never considered that the emotional response triggered by a catastrophic event could cause physical pain as well.

For years after that horrible event I worked on firefighters, first responders, and many people who had lost family and friends. The physical issues people had from working directly at Ground Zero were obvious, but to my surprise, many who hadn't been close to the site had similar problems. This terrible tragedy opened my eyes to an entirely new conundrum: pain caused by emotional stress rather than a specific physical injury. Acute trauma took on new meaning, and my understanding of how the nervous system reacts to something like 9/11 made me think differently about the brain's ability to cause a pain response.

The epiphany that shifted my hands-on practice was identifying that no matter what kind of pain or trauma a person is dealing with, the connective tissue system is the doorway into altering the nervous system and restoring balance in neurological regulation. When we're stressed, we often hear the words, "Okay, now calm down . . . it will be okay . . . don't worry." But often, that doesn't help at all. Those words can in fact make a person feel worse—like no one understands how horrible they are feeling.

What if worry and sadness are a *normal* response to a situation? Telling people not to feel that way dismisses their feelings altogether and often intensifies their stress.

Remember, pain is your brain's way of alerting you that something is off and that you need to take action. Rather than trying to quiet down the stress regulator to restore balance, I instead worked to boost the body's repair and restore regulator. The first step was getting people back into their bodies and sensing what they were feeling.

I also realized how much our personal history can dictate how we perceive pain and react to trauma in the present moment. The energy of our emotions can influence our memories, affect our current state of feeling, and make us more worried about future events. If you take an event and connect it to an emotion, it burns in your memory and you can recall it in an instant if another event triggers the same emotion. Often, this recall is unintentional and involuntary.

In other words, how you react to a current situation has some historical connection to how you reacted to something similar in the past. One interesting thing about the brain is that the regions where we process emotions, store past memories, and think about future intentions are also the regions where pain is processed.

For me, the heart of this realization was that, yes, we can rewire, repave, and reconnect our neurological wiring, especially to those areas of the body that have been neglected and are begging for our attention. What if you were constantly told as a child that you were clumsy and uncoordinated and would never make the team? How might that affect your thoughts about being a team player as an adult working in business? Or throughout your life in any situation, for that matter?

A personal example is the perception people have of me and my ability to "do anything" all by myself. The reality is, I grew up in a household where my dad told me, when I was seven: "No one wants to help you, so don't ask. If you need help and you ask for it, you'll pay a dear price, so figure it out and do it yourself. And if you can't do something yourself, then you shouldn't be doing it in the first place. When you're an adult, you won't have anyone to help you, not me or your mom, so get used to it."

That may seem harsh, and a year later when I got lost at Macy's, I became hysterical, thinking: "This is it! They left me here on purpose and I'm on my own! I don't even have a change of underwear. What do I do?" So although to the outside world I might look like an independent and capable adult—and I am—it's a forced independence. My emotional challenge is to ask for help in the face of assuming that no one will help me if I ask. And, of course, if I lose my way somewhere, I get very frustrated and anxious.

Luckily, I've had the opportunity to work with amazing mentors and therapists, and I've done a lot of soul-searching to identify my emotional triggers. I've learned that I have to exercise the choice to ask for help, and it's been amazing to consciously practice doing things differently. I've rewired my worry and fear that I'm not worth helping and instead feel thankful and grateful for any help I'm given. And when help is offered without my asking for it, well, I feel like I've won the lottery. It's a gift.

Whatever your own history, your story lives on in your cells and your nervous system, yet we often don't realize that this history is the cause of our current reactions. Can we learn to catch and stop a habitual action before we do it? Why not just reprogram the pathways and reinstate them? It doesn't matter how much of a side street your nervous system has been on—if you want to move onto the fast track of the highway, all you need is intention, specificity, and the right tools to build the road. If somebody hands you a spatula and some spackle to lay down a new road and build a foundation, it's not going to work. But if somebody gives you the right tools and the right instructions, it's easy to change your stability pathways and build a sturdy new foundation.

In fact, it's not hard to rewire the nervous system—especially if it's the peripheral nervous system that's signaling the brain to send a distress signal in the first place. Instead of trying to persuade the brain to change, why not restore the environment that the sensory nerves live in—the body's connective tissues—and send new, more solid messages back to the brain and allow the brain to adapt and make a new response? It sounds technical, and in truth it is, but restoring neurological stability is easy if you know how to do it.

Think about something that took you time to learn, like riding a bike. At first, balancing on two wheels was difficult and took a lot of mental energy. But after a bit of practice, it became much easier, and eventually habitual. Riding a bike, and every other habitual activity, follows the same behavioral and neurological patterns, starting with a three-part psychological pattern called a habit loop.

Habits are formed first by a trigger that activates a key region of the brain called the basal ganglia. This is the aspect of the autonomic nervous system that lets a behavior unfold. Then there's the routine or practice, followed by reward or success, which helps your brain remember the habit loop in the future. This area of your brain also plays a key role in the development of your emotions, memories, and pattern recognition. Although decision-making is processed in another area of the brain called your prefrontal cortex, once a behavior becomes automatic, you don't even think about it—like riding a bike. You just think about where you are going. With

NeuroStrength, you'll have to think a lot to move very little, but the reward is moving well without thinking about it.

As you learned in Chapter 1, NeuroStrength is not about muscle strength. Many people who are super-strong get injured, live with daily pain, and then feel they have to train even harder once they get better to make up for lost time. They're always trying to catch up. I often hear them say, "I just want to go back to the way things were." That, unfortunately, is the kind of attitude that will kill your future—because we can't change the past and hope for a total rewind. The past is done. The future's unknown. We've got to live in the present. Yet you have probably found yourself saying, "Oh, when I was younger, I easily ran six miles a day. I was super-fit. I was thin. It was so easy to lose weight. I was this. I was that. But life did this to me. My body is failing me."

My response to this is, *No, your body's not failing you. You're failing to listen.* Misuse, overuse, disuse, and, of course, the dreaded aging process . . . our repetitive lifestyles and choices are what cause dysfunction. So in reality, *we* are the dysfunction—not our bodies. But guess what? This is not complicated to fix—as long as you want to fix it and have the right tools to make a change! Even if your past is full of issues from injuries or trauma, the brain is a pliable system that can be reshaped no matter what you've experienced. I know you can rebuild your emotional foundation and change your functional foundation, too.

▶ Why Your Emotions Can Cause Physical Pain

In many ways, I'm grateful to pain. At the peak of my fitness career, sudden chronic pain stopped me in my tracks. I didn't figure out where this debilitating pain was coming from until years later. In my twenties I was accustomed to aches and pains caused by athleticism. I'd never considered that emotions from the past and perhaps psychic energy working to express itself could cause physical pain.

Exactly one year after my foot pain started, my father was diagnosed with terminal lung cancer and subsequently died. It may seem far-fetched to those who believe pain only comes from tissue damage, but I believe my energy body felt his energy shifting before the diagnosis. It was as if my roots were being pulled out of the dysfunctional foundation he'd created for me. I look back on those years and believe my body was asking me to take action and ground myself because something big was about to occur.

After he passed away, I explored the emotional trauma from my childhood. Almost overnight, my foot pain disappeared. This miraculous healing sent me down a path to understand what, aside from an athletic or repetitive stress injury, could cause pain to suddenly arise and become persistent. What I realized years afterward, with the help of inner reflection, therapy, and bodywork, is that there is an emotional link I'd never considered. It taught me that learning and knowledge can make you smarter, but emotions make you react and require a conscious action to create real change.

I had ignored the emotional component that was driving my behavior—the fact that I'd been living on my own for nearly a decade made no difference. I was standing on the foundation my father had created. The invisible, internal thinking that didn't reflect reality set up an inner conflict leading to physical pain.

The limbic system, often referred to as the "emotional brain," not only plays a role in our emotional responses, but it's also the region that processes movement, stores past memories, creates future intentions, and determines how we perceive pain. Our emotional state can affect our sense of pain as much as pain can affect our emotional state. Pain can hijack this region of the brain to express itself and make us take action, and our emotional state can amplify the pain experience.

The Link Between Movement and Emotions

One of the most empowering moments I've ever had was realizing just how brilliantly connected our body's nervous system and our body's fascial system are. They work with each other. As I started to understand more about connective tissue, I realized that this was a mega-missing link and related to persistent pain symptoms. I had studied anatomy. Why hadn't I been taught about the most abundant material in the body?

In addition, although specific areas of the brain are devoted to processing vision, touch, and hearing, no one specific cortical area is dedicated to pain. Neuroscientists have coined the term *pain matrix* to describe the multiple areas consistently activated during pain. The cortical and subcortical areas of our brains that create movement are the same areas where we process emotions. This is the inescapable conundrum we all face. If movement becomes chaotic or hard to do, your emotional state can then change and your stress levels increase. And if you're in a difficult place emotionally, how you move can be altered. That's why it's so hard to think clearly after you get injured or to concentrate on any kind of precise movements if you've just ended an important relationship or had a big problem at work.

Emotional posturing is a real thing, and emotional distress can cause obvious and severe postural distortions. Years ago I had a client in his mid-eighties named David. His upper back was so curved that when he'd lie down, his head remained curved forward. I asked him whether he had lost a loved one or was heartbroken over something. He told me that he was a Holocaust survivor and had experienced a lifetime of hardship. During our sessions I asked him to share some of his story, and as if he were reliving a moment in time, his tissue tightened, his breathing got short, and his eyes tracked the ceiling. Then, a shift, a deep breath, a momentary pause. "I've never told anyone how much this has affected me," he said. He went on to tell me how he had saved his own life—by leaving his brother and sister behind. "I feel like my heart broke that day," he added.

And there it was: his broken heart. The loss at the time was horrible, and his post-traumatic responses had seemed to have kept that shock. He shared how he feared for his life and how he didn't have anyone to protect him. Perhaps his tissues were still trying to protect him, even after all this time. I proposed this idea to him and he shared deep memories. As he opened up and expressed the feelings he'd never shared before, his body tension seemed to melt away, his breath moved his torso, and his neck tension relaxed. He cried. His body was still holding the fear and stress from long ago. His curved spine relaxed into the table, his head rested in my hands. When he stood up, he took a deep breath and said, "Golly, I feel taller." Sometimes our posture is a reflection of our current emotional state—or even our emotional history.

When you have an experience where your body's reaction is closely tied to pain—such as someone hurting you or an accident—the pain never quite fully leaves you. During that experience, your brain sent signals to your nerves and muscles, telling them how to respond. If a memory of this pain comes back to you, it can become a form of post-traumatic stress disorder, as if you were reliving the moment. Yet in working with people like David, I realized that much of our memory isn't stored in our brain alone. We store it in our *fascia*. With the right touch, and the right intention, we can call up those memories just by treating our connective tissues.

Another client, a well-known and successful professional athlete, came to me for help with knee problems and shoulder pain. During our first session as I was working on him, I asked, "Did you have braces on your legs when you were a kid?"

I could feel him stiffen in surprise, and he said, "Yes, I did, for four years because my legs were really bowed. How did you know?"

"Well, it's hard to explain how I know, but your tissues told me so," I replied. "So let's see if we can just unwind some of this old tissue."

As the session continued, he suddenly started talking about old memories, especially about being picked on by the other kids and mocked for needing braces. I told him to keep talking about it, as that was the best way to unravel in his body the fear and tension from those long-ago incidents and memories. Expressing your emotions can free your tissues of their possession.

Somato-Emotional Release

What this athlete went through is called somato-emotional release, and it's a phenomenon well-known to those who do hands-on bodywork. It can also occur when doing mindful practices such as meditation or yoga, where certain poses can trigger long-suppressed memories. I am living proof of the power of somato-emotional release. Once, a friend's dog jumped up as I bent down to pet her, and her skull and my nose collided. For a week I couldn't feel my upper lip or teeth, so another friend insisted I see Barbara Chang, an advanced craniosacral therapist. My friend had told me about this type of therapy before, but it sounded farfetched to me as a therapeutic practice.

During our first session, Barbara was working on my nose, with a very light touch. I'd never experienced anything like it. She mentioned that the left side of my nose was displaced—and in the next moment I made an audible sound and my eyes popped open.

"What was that?" Barbara said.

"Gosh, a memory just popped into my head like I just relived it."

"Tell me what you saw," she said as she continued to work.

"Well, it was just before a big softball game, and the coach did a windmill with the ball and chucked it straight at me, hard and fast. I wasn't ready for it. I tried to shield my face with my mitt, but the ball tipped the top of the glove and hit me smack dead in the bridge of my nose, so hard that it knocked me out. The next thing I knew, my dad was standing over me, with the sun behind him so I could only make him out in silhouette. Then he reached down, put his fingers on my nose, and pushed it back into place. I screamed in shock and pain, and he put his fingers up to his cigarette, took a drag, said, 'Don't worry, it'll build character,' then walked away. My nose stayed swollen for a long time. Boy, did I get picked on after that! Everybody at school was, like, 'Oh, Sue and her nose are coming to the party.' So I guess my dad was right—it *did* build character, but not in a way that was good for me."

"That's what we call a somato-emotional release," Barbara told me. "We can't hold memories just in our brain, so we store them in our tissues. Sometimes a memory calls itself back into our consciousness when we are ready to let it go and process what's in there."

I'd never heard of such a thing, but when I left her office, my nose felt a lot better and I could feel my front teeth again. What was far more bizarre, however, was that the next morning my foot didn't hurt as much. I didn't know it yet, but that was the turning point after nearly two years of debilitating pain that had forced me out of the fitness career I loved. But I was still bewildered, as Barbara hadn't gone anywhere near my foot. Maybe it was just a coincidence. Another day went by, then another, and my foot continued to improve. I called Barbara and asked her what muscle she'd been working on, because my foot was so much better.

"It wasn't a muscle," she explained. "I worked on your cranial rhythm and the bones of your skull to try to restore some balance in your body. And if I may say this, your foot problem doesn't seem like a foot problem. The thing that came to my mind when I was working on you was that you were like a little flower that somebody had grabbed at its stem and ripped up from the earth."

"That's exactly what it feels like, Barbara," I said. I was quiet for a while, and then I asked what she'd done with the cranial rhythm. "Are you saying you actually influenced the cerebrospinal fluid in my body?"

I had studied anatomy and physiology; I knew what cerebrospinal fluid was and how it fluctuated in the intercranial membranes and my spine. But I wasn't sure I knew anything about manipulating it. And even if you could, what changes could that possibly make?

"Can you feel the rhythm?" Barbara asked me. "What else can you feel?" I then shared with her how I could sense the motility of organs, restrictions in a person's diaphragmatic motion, and muscles that aren't firing properly. But how did she know what to do with what she felt? She simply said, "You know, Sue, not everyone can feel those types of things. Why don't you take a hands-on course and learn about what you can do to change people?"

So I did. I embarked on yet another transition, believing that to help restore function to a body, there was way more to treat beyond muscle balance and alignment. From basic craniosacral therapy to advanced levels of visceral manipulation, somato-emotional release, lymphatic drainage, and bioenergetics, I took every course I could. The one common thread of all of these therapeutic interventions was *fascia*. For the first time, light touch resonated beyond just palpating tissue for stiffness or lack of mobility or sensitivity. I felt I could transform a person back to ideal function in a unique way.

Despite the fact that these techniques helped my clients, I still struggled to find scientific evidence and research papers on the techniques I was using. My desire to gain more understanding of the results I witnessed sent me down the neurofascial rabbit hole from which I've never returned. Now, years later, I am a founding member of the Fascia Research Society, and have worked to create research studies to measure changes in fascia as it relates to functional improvements. The leaders of this society founded the Fascia Research Congress, which continues to bring researchers and clinicians together to promote collaboration and bring research to the forefront of the therapeutic and biological fields of human science.

▶ How the Past Shapes Your Present

"I don't want to talk about it. Why does it matter anyway?" So many people say this when asked about their past. They often live their whole lives without addressing the painful experiences that shaped them—not realizing, as I didn't for many years, what effect holding on to these experiences, most often unconsciously, has on their nervous system.

Your nervous system, as you learned already, is designed to support, protect, and stabilize you, to keep you alive and to sustain homeostasis. Even after a drug addict injects a drug that could kill him or her, that addict's nervous system doesn't give in without a fight. It will continue to try to support, protect, and stabilize the addict's body even in the face of such deliberate injury.

In addition, many people don't realize that their fascia is the environment in which everything in the body lives; and without a doubt, our environments—interior and exterior—have a significant effect on how we function and sustain our resilience. Intelligence is only partly based on DNA. If a genius child isn't raised in a family environment that supports his or her brilliant mind, that child is less likely to become an Albert Einstein or a Marie Curie. Our environments matter.

I learned this through my own personal experiences. I've been lucky enough in my adult life to have found a unique psychologist who helped me realize how my personal history was linked to how I reacted to people or situations. I, too, had never considered how often I react to a current situation because of the habitual reactions and responses I innately possess from my past.

Undoing the Power of the Thought Virus

Evolutionary biologist Richard Dawkins coined the word *meme* in his 1976 book *The Selfish Gene*. He described a meme as a type of contagious information, something like fashion or a catchphrase that propagates itself. Although he was talking about genes and how we pass information to our offspring before they're even born, this occurs in our lives all the time as ideas, comments, or beliefs are passed from person to person or brain to brain. What are often called thought viruses can be processed and stored in the brain. With the billions of bits of information our brain receives, storing this information for later use is just a part of our brain's process.

Here's a simple example of a thought virus. When I was twelve, I hurt my knee while playing soccer. After the doctor treated me, my mother said, "You're going to have a bad knee just like me." That comment set a thought virus into my head. Although I soon forgot about this injury, when I reinjured my knee playing soccer a few years later, I thought, "My knee is getting worse and it's going to be all messed up like my mother's knee." Here was that thought virus rearing its ugly head years later.

Fast-forward to when I was twenty-two and teaching aerobics. My knee started hurting again—because I'd been teaching almost thirty aerobic classes every week. My knee was buckling out from under me at random moments, and again I thought, "Wow, something is really wrong. My knee is just like my mom's. She was right!" A doctor told me that I'd torn my meniscus in three places, and my only choice was surgical removal.

My mother had also told me why her knee was so bad. One day she fell off her bike and cracked her kneecap. The pain got so bad that her mom took her to the doctor, and they removed part of her kneecap. She was confined to a wheelchair and sent to live with the nuns at a children's hospital for almost four months. She told me that having surgery was the worst thing she'd ever gone through and she hoped she'd never have to go through it again.

This was another thought virus for me. But this one turned out to be a good one, because when the doctor told me they had to remove my meniscus, I said, "No, I think I'll keep it." The surgeon looked at me, perplexed, and said, "You can't keep it. It won't repair and will only get worse."

"It's my knee, so actually, I *can* keep it," I told him flatly.

"If you don't get the surgery, you'll walk with a permanent limp by the time you're thirty," he barked back.

"I came here to find out what was wrong with my knee, and now I know, and I think I can fix it," I told him. And then the thought virus added, "If I have this knee surgery, then I'll be just like my mom."

So I worked with Jim and Phil Wharton who trained me in a technique called Active Isolated Stretching, created by Aaron Mattes. I learned that weak hip stabilizers and other imbalances were causing the repetitive strain on my knee. I trained to heal my knee for eight months and wore a splint while still teaching classes every week to pay my bills. A year later, my knee stopped hurting. And now, nearly three decades later, my knee never hurts at all. I reprogrammed my brain, shifted my thought virus, and today I can adamantly say, *My knee is not just like my mother's.*

Thoughts are incredibly powerful. Usually, if something hurts, we go to a doctor. If a doctor can't find something specifically wrong, we can become frustrated. Some of my clients say, "If a doctor can't figure this out, something must be *really* wrong." That, too, is a thought virus if the reason you feel that way is because at some point in the past there was an unsolvable problem that no one could figure out and that experience ingrained itself into your nervous system. We form beliefs about something and we can't get those beliefs out of our heads. From behavior to capabilities, identity, and values, our brains have interesting ways of reactivating thought viruses formed by memories from long ago. It often takes a good therapist or friend to help a person recognize the patterns.

For example, when I was in my early thirties, I took up skydiving. On my fortieth jump my chute strings became entangled, sending me into an uncontrolled spin. Although I managed to untangle myself and regain control, every time I went to jump after that, I would relive that moment and the thought virus would tell me, "It might happen again." After another dozen jumps, I couldn't shake that viral fear, which stopped me from enjoying jumping anymore, so I stopped. The exhilaration and joy I once felt hurling myself into the air made me sick to my stomach. Thought viruses can truly make you feel sick, even though, it's all just in your mind . . . or is it?

This happens with athletes, too. An injury, and the related thought viruses *This could happen again* or *This could ruin my career,* can stop a person from playing a sport because of the fear of further damage or having their entire life and future compromised permanently from the chances of a reoccurring injury.

Neurons That Fire Together, Wire Together

One of the reasons why thought viruses can form is our brain's powerful ability to store information for later use. This is one aspect of neuroplasticity (discussed in Chapter 1). The saying "neurons that fire together, wire together" was coined by neuropsychologist Donald Hebb in 1949. His work in the field of associative learning led to the understanding that every experience, thought, feeling, and sensation triggers thousands of neurons, which form a neural network. If we repeat an experience enough times, our brain learns to trigger the same neurons each time.

These neural networks can have positive or negative effects. In a positive way, they can help us learn, memorize, and recall information very effectively. Neural networks allow baseball players to accurately hit a ball without having to think about how to swing the bat. But a neural network can also go awry. A tragic example would be a child who has suffered abuse. Physical contact of any kind—even a simple hug— might be enough to trigger a fight-or-flight response. The child's body may pull back or jump merely from the thought of being touched. This is the root of post-traumatic stress disorder, or PTSD.

An athletic example would be a cyclist who had an accident when her wheels went over the yellow lines on a downhill turn, causing them to slip out from under her. Long after that accident, when she goes down a steep hill, her brain is working to avoid those lines, her body becomes stiffer, she may even put her brakes on to "avoid another accident." Yet these reactions can in fact cause an accident, and over time, other types of pain from involuntary reactions, such as prolonged shoulder tension leading to neck pain.

Pain is based on your brain's perceptions of a possible threat, and your brain always produces your sense of pain.

Jan walked into my office with neck pain and carpal tunnel syndrome, which is a painful condition of the hand and fingers caused by repetitive movements over a long period or by fluid retention. It is characterized by sensations of tingling, numbness, or burning. Her doctor told her that it can't be fixed without surgery.

During my intake, I asked about her job, and her body instantly became tense and looked uncomfortable. She squirmed as she described frustrations at work, and her hands clenched into fists and her voice elevated in tone. This type of physical reaction isn't uncommon—but we don't realize that *we* are the cause of our dysfunction, not *our job*. It's our reactions to our environment that cause physical issues.

I explained this to Jan, and she told me her neck pain increases the second she walks into her office and hears her boss's voice. "I can't stand the way he smells," she said, "and his voice sounds like my ex-husband, whom I despise."

There it was—the dysfunctional emotional cascade that causes actual, medically diagnosable symptoms, which Jan's doctor recommended surgery to fix. But the source of her pain was her feelings about her ex-husband, triggered by a boss who smelled and sounded like him. No wonder her neck was stiff and her hands numb. She was clenching every aspect of her being, choking her voice of expression, and living in an energy like the one she had broken free of.

When people tie themselves to pain, it also becomes their thought virus. The thought virus worms its way in and they tells them that they can't get better until a doctor diagnoses them. Often, they're so paralyzed with fear that they won't even go to a doctor.

Why do we hold on to certain memories? Are they serving a purpose? How often do you find yourself reliving a bad memory? I'll bet you do that more often than you relive a good memory. Yes, it's cathartic to talk about something, but at the same time, it's much more common for the thought virus to take over. In fact, the more you talk about a particular incident in a negative way, the more that memory is rewired so you never forget it.

This is a very hard idea for people to understand, because we all know how difficult it can be to talk about emotions. I've seen this time and again with athletes whose career is on the line when they get injured. They have no choice but to get quick-fix surgery, as their coaches and team need them back out on the field as fast as possible. Often, this sends these athletes into even more of a tailspin, as they aren't allowed to address the underlying causes of their pain.

One semi-pro baseball player came to see me with severe neck pain he'd had for months. I asked him to tell me about his family, and he told me about his mother's recent heart attack and other worrisome issues. "Gosh, that's an awful lot for you to deal with right now," I told him. "Are you talking to anybody?"

"I can't," he said. "God forbid anyone starts knowing about it. I'll lose my first line position, and I'm trying to go pro. How do I get around that?"

We are so often trained to deal with our emotions by *not* dealing with them.

By keeping them quiet. Keeping them under cover. Not talking about them. We're supposed to stuff our emotions down and just get on with things.

No wonder our bodies have had enough!

"What Hurts You Will Make You Stronger" Is a Fallacy

I was walking down that same road, so I sat down with a therapist after my dad died and shared some of the most painful incidents I had experienced with him. I added that whenever I talked about him with my friends, their response was almost always, "Oh, he was just trying to make you stronger." Actually, I already knew that he hadn't been doing that, but this notion had been said to me so often that I started making excuses, explaining to the therapist that my dad had had his own horrible childhood and was just mirroring his own experiences to me, and that maybe it wasn't about me at all.

The therapist sat there for a moment and then said: "Actually, your father sounds sadistic. No wonder you're feeling horrible. Of course you should feel that way. I would feel that way, too, if somebody said things like that to me. Do you really think he was trying to make you stronger? What do you think he was doing?"

This blew my mind. "I think he was trying to undermine my gifts," I said eventually, "because I think they scared him."

The therapist nodded. "I think so, too. I think you scared him to death. Now that sounds a whole lot more like reality than the other thing."

"Can I actually say that out loud?" I wondered.

"You should say that as your mantra, Sue," he replied. "You had something, and it's scary for a parent to see their kid have something special. And sometimes parents want to control their children's lives. In fact, what they think and how they act might not even have anything to do with you. It's about their own fears, and their own issues, and that's the thing we take on."

I thought hard about those words. Perhaps it was okay to be so angry about how I was treated rather than feeling bad about feeling angry. I was able to unravel so much of the fear that had been instilled in me. After my father died, I came to understand that I could rewrite my history to be the person that I was born to be, rather than the person I was told I *had* to be. I was able to rebuild myself into a new person. The pain in my foot never came back. If something hurt—perhaps my neck was stiff after a long flight—I'd go home, MELT for a while, eat a good dinner, get a good night's sleep, and wake up with no pain.

In other words, I took good care of myself. I still do. I eat well, I get massages, I run, I meditate, I talk, I think, I express—and I do my best to not let negative energy fester. After a decade of therapy, I was more able to ask myself why I acted certain ways and to assess how my damaging childhood affected my adult choices. Don't get me wrong, the challenges of my history still affect me and my life today, but I'm more aware of that and I work to not let it hold me back from being my true self.

Which brings me back to what I said at the beginning of this chapter: *emotions make you react*. They're a big deal. Yet we're taught to mask all the problems and look for a solution to the symptoms, not the root of the problems.

Sometimes we just need to be very quiet with our bodies and say these words: "I'm sorry. Please forgive me. I love you. I'm sorry I've been gone so long, but now that I'm back, I promise I'll stay."

Say that to your inner child, inner warrior, inner king, inner queen. Whenever I delve into this topic during my trainings, many eyes start to well up with tears. It is deeply cathartic for me to see how addressing thought viruses makes enormous changes to a person's psyche. Learning how to express your emotions without negative consequences takes practice. But once you can do this, it allows you to identify and work on true transformation, and those tears are an invitation for you to go deeper. It's okay to recognize those emotions and to grow, and to change, and to learn. If you try to keep thought viruses buried, chances are high that they will rise to the surface when they are least expected—and certainly not wanted.

▶ Treating Trauma

Traumatic events happen. If they aren't happening to you personally, you hear about them all around you. We tend to think of trauma in terms of one-time incidents, such as another school shooting or a terrorist bombing, but trauma can also become an emotional and ongoing issue, such as having to live in an abusive household or losing your job or a loved one.

We all manage trauma in basically two ways. The first is the state of hyperarousal—you can't calm down, your brain races, you can't fall asleep or stay asleep because you keep replaying the trauma such that it disrupts your attention and focus. The second way is the state of numbness—a sense of tuning out and a constant feeling of lethargy. A total shutdown of the senses can also happen because of what trauma does to the mind.

One of the most powerful things I've done during my years as a hands-on therapist is instill hope in clients when their nervous systems' response to trauma was either to shut down or to stir them up so high they couldn't think straight. It's important (and helpful) to know that recovering from trauma is a survival mechanism we are all equipped with.

Our nervous system manages stress automatically. We all have a "fight, flight, or freeze" response that occurs without our awareness or control. This response is a remnant of our evolutionary history, when constant physical danger was lurking. We often don't realize this response is happening, nor do we know why we instantly react the way we do. Usually, our immediate reactions are created on the basis of previous traumatic events that we may have consciously forgotten.

When something traumatic happens, what do you do? Who do you talk to? Usually, the fight, flight, or freeze response happens first—coming from the reptilian part of the brain—and then social engagement comes later. People commiserate to manage stress; you see this happening on social media all the time. Getting others to engage in our feelings makes us feel less alone in the fear and trauma that we have experienced—whether the trauma actually happened to us, we witnessed it, or we heard it on the news. Our brain often doesn't even know the difference.

The Past Is the Past

As I've mentioned, my clients constantly say, "I just want to go back to the way things were. I want my old life back." Well, sorry, that can't happen. And what's worse, sometimes the past makes thinking of the future more miserable than it actually might turn out to be. We can't predict the future. We can take a pretty good guess about it, but the actions we take today are what are going to shape tomorrow.

Our actions and desires sometimes don't mesh, and the reason we act this way says a *lot* about our past, more than it does about the present. Sometimes we talk ourselves into reasons we can't get what we want or we can't have the life we want because in reality we don't know what we want in the first place. It becomes easier to blame problems on something we think is unfixable rather than tackling them head-on. It's a vicious cycle that many people find themselves in after a trauma.

What makes it even trickier is that people usually feel a kind of shame after trauma. Not only do they suffer from their hyperarousal or numbness, but from their *thoughts* because they feel terrible about their emotions. But why *wouldn't* a person feel that way after trauma? They were a victim of something they can't take back. The feeling of helplessness can certainly be hardwired in the deep regions of the brain where we process emotions, actions, past occurrences, and even future intentions.

Shifting Physiology and Behavior

Often I find in trauma that it's not that the stress response of the brain is too high, it's that the rest and repair aspects are shut down. The *repair* response rather than the stress response is the real issue. A person can become dissociated from their conscious ability to shift their traumatized state of mind, which is tough to do on one's own. That's one reason self-care isn't intuitive or used by those who suffer from trauma or PTSD, even though it's the best thing for it, as long as they get proper guidance.

This is why the MELT Rebalance Sequence has such a powerful effect on PTSD. A simple technique called the 3-D Breath Breakdown focuses on inhalation to arouse the sympathetic aspects of the nervous system. Although breathing is autonomic and involuntary, we can consciously control it if we want to. And when we do so, we intervene in the sympathetic response. Then by activating the neurological core reflex on an exhale, we boost parasympathetic tone and improve overall regulation.

▶ Building a Sturdy Emotional Foundation

You can go to all the trainings and classes in the world, but if you've built your emotional foundation on something that's not sturdy, you're never going to get maximum results.

The goal is to achieve your personal best, not to compare yourself to anyone else. That's what athletes do, and it's like psychological terrorism inside their heads that leads to envy, anger, and frustration. If you're angry that you're not as good as someone else, it's easier to hold on to that feeling than to deal with the emotional justification behind your behavior.

Our history lays down an emotional foundation where we root our beliefs. Our beliefs can drive us and compel us in negative ways, to eating disorders, overworking, and overexercising, or in a positive ways, to good health, happiness, and balance.

Beliefs can influence our identity—because if you don't believe in yourself to begin with, you're never going to achieve your goals or full potential.

People who achieve something extraordinary, whatever they do, believe that they're good at what they do. Without that belief, it's almost impossible to succeed. How do you turn your beliefs into reality to give you the positive results you seek?

The Power of Unconditional Love and Support

As an adult, I can now recognize that my parents could have been more supportive when I was growing up instead of using psychological terrorism and harsh punishments. When I was young, I didn't consider their actions and words "abusive" because I thought that all kids grew up in a household like mine. If anything, I always blamed myself.

So I needed to repattern my neurological system once I grew up because I didn't feel that I'd been given the unconditional love and support I believe every child deserves. My dad consistently told me why my ideas were wrong—it was his way or the highway. He also didn't like me to do things without his permission and put the fear of God in me if I did, so I learned to be quiet and fly under the radar. My mom didn't speak up about this because she was getting the same message. So I internalized it, thinking that I was somehow bad; but I still remember a day, when I was about ten, when I looked in the mirror and said to myself: *He's wrong. I am special. I'm a good person.*

This shaky emotional foundation created a conflict between my internal sense of self and the external bullying by my father—I was living in a constant state of fight or flight. It wasn't until after my dad died that the conflict lifted. I recall singing, "Ding dong, the witch is dead . . . the wicked witch is dead!" and feeling a sense of freedom.

Perhaps the main reason that I survived my childhood to create MELT and become a healthy, happily functioning adult was that I had one person in my young life—my beloved great-grandmother—who gave me the support I needed. One day, she asked me why I was sitting with her and not out playing with the kids. I told her I didn't fit in, that I was weird, and that the other kids didn't like me. She asked me who had said I was weird, and I told her my dad had—all the time. I also said that sometimes I felt and thought things that my dad said weren't normal, and he said that I'd scare people so I had to stop feeling and thinking them. My great-grandmother told me that I wasn't weird and that, instead, I had a gift. "What you think is a curse today might be your greatest blessing," she added. "Don't lose it, just keep it to yourself. It will come to you—why you can do what you do. You *are* full of love."

She gave me the validation I needed to push past my hurt. I don't know how she knew what she knew. She was special to me and had the gift of being so full of love that I felt safe. You need just one person to give you unconditional support and love. My great-grandmother was that person. She gave me hope.

If you didn't have that one person in your life, it's never too late to give *yourself* the love you need. And although we may never meet face to face, I'm giving you unconditional love and support. I believe you have in you the ability to heal yourself and find balance even in a world that may seem out of control, chaotic, and ungrounded.

▶ Strengthening Your Emotional Resilience

What is resilience? For me, resilience represents vitality, integrity, power, and connection, and a positive sense of feeling and moving effortlessly with control. It's having adaptability, being open to more than one choice, and moving forward even when faced with setbacks.

Many of us tell ourselves that if a problem is hard to get rid of, we have every right to hold on to the problem instead of trying to solve it and end it. So, the question is, do you want to heal or not? Change is more possible if you believe change can happen.

The whole point of NeuroStrength is to say to yourself: *My body has the ability to heal; it's just lost its way. I have the ability to reroute myself away from the path of least resistance. I'm going to make new pathways. I'm going to figure it out as I go. I'm going to take that risk. I might be scared. I might fail fifty more times, but I'll keep trying. I'm worth it.*

Just like a baby getting up on all fours for the first time—it takes a lot of attempts before that happens. But once they get up, they do that rocking thing. They start looking around for everybody else to notice, as if they're saying: *OMG! Are you guys seeing what I'm doing? Isn't this incredible? Look at me! I got this!*

Where does that innate resilience, the living embodiment of neurological stability, go? That baby is pure resilience, because the resilience is what gets him or her to try again to get up on all fours, ready to conquer the world. Don't focus on how many tries it takes; focus on the outcome you want to achieve. This is what will restore your innate resilience.

Feels Like the First Time

When I used to play softball, sometimes the second the ball was out of the pitcher's hand, I knew I was going to crush it. Athletes understand this. How do they *know*? Because they're "in the zone," and all of the energy is right on their primal pathways. I think that's why athletes get so elated when they're in the zone and they score; this emotional response is imprinted in the same parts of the brain that were stimulated when we crawled or walked for the first time. It's like the first time all over again.

That's what you're striving for, because the first time you achieve something will always make you happy. Every time the baseball player hears that sweet sound of nailing the ball, it's like a first-ever home run. This is why being a fan is just as exciting as being an athlete—every time a home run is hit, it's as if *you* did it yourself for the first time, too. You're celebrating as part of the tribe.

When you find your tribe, the connection reinforces your internal, emotional resilience. I hope you'll be able to meld together the physical resilience that MELT Performance gives you with the emotional resilience it helps you develop. Of course, this isn't likely to happen every day—some days are awful, and some are incomparable, but most are somewhere in the middle. That's just life!

That's where MELT comes in. We reconnect and tune in to what might be the actual lurking problems that we don't see, and then we rebalance the foundation. We rehydrate and nurture. We make sure that the environment is healthy and thriving. Then we release the compression in those spaces, so that now we can reintegrate the neurological timing of our pelvis and shoulders, and then we can repattern these movements.

Once you've got a new foundation, you can rebuild your strength all you want. You'll use your new understanding of stability and the NeuroStrength techniques to continue to rebuild more and more, to reach new goals. In fact, you might surprise yourself as to what achievements you can reach when stability becomes your new norm.

If you earned a million dollars one year, your new goal may be to see whether you can hit two million. You don't stop. You always look forward. You walk down the street with your eyes on the horizon, rather than walking down the street with your eyes lowered. If you don't look around every once in a while, you could miss the most amazing sights, right in front of you.

NeuroStrength is a combination of your neurological stability and all of your emotional experience. It's you bringing the excitement and the kind of mental juice you get from doing something the first time. When you have a bad day and your emotions cloud reality, NeuroStrength allows you to check in on the engine of your neurological system, add some new oil, maybe do some tweaking and tuning, and consider that what's going on is sometimes out of your control.

Change Your Mind, Change Your Body

Change is tough. Our bodies resist change, too—they take the path of least resistance, as you saw in Chapter 1. Not only is change tough, but it's uncomfortable. We grasp on to those old, worn-out beliefs that do not serve our current desires. The shift in my understanding caused by my foot pain was a true moment of change that set me on a path to help others live pain-free and reconnect to their body's true potential of optimal function.

If I had known about MELT when I was a competitive athlete, I wouldn't have been filled with fear that I would never be good enough because, like all of my colleagues, I was constantly getting injured. That is a bad fear to possess as an athlete, because fear gets in the way of performance. Fear gets in the way of *everything*!

I am no longer afraid. I have an incredible business and am surrounded by love. I am no longer ruled by the trauma of my childhood. At forty-eight, I look more vibrant than I did twenty years ago. I feel blessed that I learned how to fix my pain and my health in my twenties, because the tangible results are so obvious two decades later. I even had more wrinkles then than I do now!

That's why when people ask me, "How long will the changes last?," I always say, "The question you should be asking is, how little time can I devote to myself in a day to create lasting changes that will make tomorrow even better?" A little self-care goes a long way if you know how to do it well.

In my years as a teacher and hands-on bodyworker, I've learned that one of the greatest gifts I can give people is a belief in their resilience and the hope and self-empowerment to restore it. Resilience means that no matter what is thrown at you, you effortlessly cope with it rather than bottling it up in your body like a ticking time bomb. Why wait for pain signals to take action when you can rewire your neural pathways, become more stable, and therefore stronger and more resilient? The sooner you start, the sooner in your life you'll harness your youthful, vibrant energy. When you have a core belief in your resilience, you will always be moving forward.

The resilience that you will develop using the techniques in this book is profound. If you're not feeling good, you're going to feel better; and if you're already feeling good, then you're going to stay that way. It's you telling your body that you aren't giving up. You might be in pain. You might think you can't do it. You might never have moved your body in these ways before. But I'm here to say that *anybody* can do this—at any age and any fitness level.

PART TWO

The Foundation of NeuroStrength Moves

4

A MELT Method Refresher
The Four Rs of the MELT Protocol

As I wrote in *The MELT Method*, the secret to living the pain-free life you deserve is rehydrating your connective tissue and restoring balance in the three regulators I discussed in Chapter 2 through the Four Rs of MELT: Reconnect, Rebalance, Rehydrate, and Release. This is the foundation of self-care and hands-off bodywork. This chapter presents a short primer/refresher on the concepts that make MELT so effective. Many of the moves and sequences in MELT are the foundation of MELT Performance, so it's important that you understand the concepts and know how to do the basics.

When it comes to aches and pain, we focus on the areas that hurt. If our neck aches, we want someone to dig a ball or a fist into our neck and press as hard as possible to make the ache stop. But the reality is, we focus so much on the painful areas, we don't take a moment to understand what's causing the pain in the first place. It's like beating up a victim instead of searching for the perpetrator causing the victim to cry out for help.

With MELT, you learn simple assessment techniques to reconnect you to what's really going on. This helps you figure out where the accumulated stuck stress is in your body that's causing your pain—rather than focusing on the pain itself. The Rebalance techniques help our body manage stress, repair, and improve digestion by accessing the diaphragm and the intrinsic aspects of our core stability. Next, you rehydrate the environment that everything lives in, which is your connective tissue. Finally, you release the spaces or joints where you feel compressed and tense. When you add in the NeuroStrength techniques, you will reintegrate the neurological mechanisms that stabilize your pelvis and shoulder girdle as well as the timing and sensorimotor control of your NeuroCore. Once you have better stability, you repattern primary movement patterns to improve your overall function. After that, you will be able to rebuild your strength, agility, and overall stamina and power. You can get stronger without compensation accumulating and causing dysfunction and poor movement patterns. You can achieve body goals that you never could before, because you will have established the firm foundation your body truly needs.

▶ The Neurofascial Cascade of Dysfunction

Your brain is constantly sending you messages, but are you listening? Have you ever felt a little stiff when you stood up after sitting for a long time? Or have your feet or back ever felt achy when you get out of bed in the morning? These aches and stiffness are so common we never think they're a problem because when you move around they seem to subside. As you recall, these are what I call *pre-pain signals*.

Like a slow-moving river, daily living creates and deposits sediment that alters the river's natural flow. As that sediment accumulates, the end result is what I call stuck stress. Once it starts accumulating, stuck stress causes even more symptoms. What starts off as a pre-pain signal can quickly change into a persistent state of joint pain and muscle ache, as well as lead to a decline in your overall performance. The adaptations on a cellular and neurological level can be catastrophic.

If you do what most people do, ignore these signals or take ibuprofen to tone down the pain, you start having symptoms that seem completely unrelated to connective tissue issues—things like sudden weight gain, trouble digesting food, or difficulty concentrating. As tired as you might feel during the day, when you try to fall asleep at night, you can't. Or you wake up in the middle of the night and can't fall back asleep. Are these symptoms sounding familiar?

Now you have a bigger problem since most of your body's natural healing and repair processes occur during deep sleep. If your sleep isn't restorative, your body's natural repair mechanisms can't do their job, and you wake up the next morning with a backlog of stress. Metabolic waste accumulates, low-grade inflammation occurs, and hormones and neurotransmitters go haywire. Autonomic regulation gets out of balance, your lymphatic system becomes compromised, and you are now increasing your chances of an autoimmune deregulation. Not only do you feel "not quite right," but all of these things can lead to depression, anxiety, and what most people would consider the negative effects of aging.

We can't stop the aging process, but many of the unwanted effects of it are avoidable or reversible, especially through effective self-care treatments like MELT.

Although sipping water regularly and eating water-filled foods is essential to your overall good health, when connective tissue loses its adaptability, your cells don't absorb water or nutrients efficiently and the pre-lymphatic system gets bogged down like a traffic jam on a highway. Likewise, changing your diet, exercising more, or sleeping in on weekends doesn't make a dent in your stuck stress. As important as daily activity and a healthy diet are, they don't directly address the issue in your connective tissue, and no pill or surgery can fix it, but MELTing has been designed to do just that.

Although your brain produces your perception of pain, I always say, "If aches and pain are persistent, there's an issue in your connective tissue—it's not just in your mind." This is the foundation of the MELT Method, and it's critical to your overall performance.

◗ The Living Body Model

When I started teaching the MELT Method, I had to simplify the terminology to make the concepts easier to understand and implement. I coined the phrase *Living Body Model* to express the involuntary aspects of neurofascial function. This model has five elements focused on the autonomic aspects of healthy living, allowing you to assess and practice self-care in a manner that is applicable to human beings rather than anatomical models. You'll see these terms used in the MELT moves and sequences.

AUTOPILOT: The parts of your body that protect, support, and stabilize you without your voluntary control or conscious awareness.

BODY SENSE: There are two aspects of Body Sense—one is learning to tune in to our own body during self-assessment to identify common imbalances; the other is learning to understand that our own body does something similar for us without our conscious knowledge or control. Within the nervous system there are receptors that sense this positioning, and the two primary ones are called proprioceptors and interoceptors. The Autopilot uses these like a GPS system. It monitors the position of our joints in relationship to gravity so movements are precise while overseeing and managing our physiological condition. Learning to consciously use Body Sense instead of our common senses like touch or vision to identify common imbalances is the foundation of MELT's self-care assessments; change occurs when we create a new connection to how we sense what we feel within our body.

MASSES AND SPACES: A structural assessment tool so you don't have to know anatomy. Masses and spaces are used as reference points in all of the MELT moves to identify proper body position and placement. Our primary masses are the head, ribs, and pelvis. The primary spaces are the neck and low back.

NEUROCORE: A simplified term to describe the involuntary neurological mechanisms and reflexes and sensorimotor function that give us inherent stability without our conscious control. The deep core or central reflexes that stabilize the masses and spaces (most specifically the pelvis and spine) and protect the organs is what I call the Reflexive Core Mechanism. The ground reaction forces we use to sustain upright joint positioning and the reflexes that keep our brain connected to our center of gravity to stop us from falling down is what I call the Rooted Core Mechanism. When the NeuroCore functions efficiently, our body feels grounded, movement feels effortless, and our masses remain stable over our feet.

TENSIONAL ENERGY: Mechanical pressure, stretch, and vibration (where breathing is one form of vibration) create neurochemical changes in the body called mechanotransduction. When mechanotransduction occurs, the collagen within fascia acts like a superconductor allowing cell-to-cell and structure-to-structure communication to occur, and the resulting fluid flow generates consistent movement from fascia to lymph structures. *Tensional energy* is a dynamic term that simplifies these concepts and gives importance to enhancing the fluid components and spaces between the fascial fibers to increase our body's mobility and stability. The mechanical compression and lengthening techniques called Rehydrate moves are designed to improve the mobility and integrity of this system as a way to create better joint alignment, mobility, and muscular flexibility.

▶ The Science Behind the Living Body Model

When I alleviated my own pain using light-touch therapeutic intervention, I was amazed that it worked, but I wanted to understand *why* it worked. What I discovered was that most of these techniques did not yet have a lot of scientific evidence to support them. Just because someone claims something doesn't make it a fact. That a technique "normalizes the frequencies of neurons" or "regulates the natural rhythms of the body" sounds great, but how are these changes measured? Most therapies consider clinical examinations and clients' subjective responses as valid measurements of change, but can we explain what really caused these changes? There's not necessarily anything wrong with those theories—the fact is that many of the modalities I've studied really do make profound changes even without science explicitly defining what's happening. I'm sure other practitioners would agree: If we waited for double-blind, peer-reviewed research to validate therapeutic results, we'd never help anyone. Fortunately, science is catching up to clinical evidence and continues to refine what I understand about longevity and harnessing resilience. I created MELT to be as evidence-based as possible, and I continue to seek new evidence to explain how MELT works and how it can work even better and also to develop new research using the method.

Twenty years ago I thought that the connective tissue and autonomic nervous systems were as separate as the digestive and skeletal systems. Today more than ever, I am beginning to comprehend just how interconnected and interdependent our internal systems truly are. Plus, I have a mild obsession with reading research papers. The internet was just emerging when I started seeking answers and my access to research papers was limited. Today, *PubMed*, *Research Gate*, the *Journal of Bodywork and Manual Therapy*, the National Institutes of Health, and other respected organizations are online making resources easily available to clinicians. I'm also just an email away from the top researchers to ask questions directly. I know the folly of confirmation bias, and I'm committed to ongoing research because the more answers I get the more questions I have. Every time I read a research paper I realize how much I don't know. It's as if learning comes with its own guarantee of continual learning, leading to the never-ending joy of exploration.

My passion and mission for MELT was, and still is, to uncover and simplify neurofascial science in a way that empowers the general public without overwhelming them with the jargon from multiple disciplines that results in a sense of separation and helplessness. My goal is to find and uphold the necessary, fascia-like, tensional, relationship boundary between clinical outcomes, theory, and valid science.

▶ International Fascia Research Congress

I've been privileged to be a founding member of the Fascia Research Society. Since its inception, over a decade ago, the scientists, researchers, and clinicians I've been able to connect with have shared their work and expertise with me, helped me to develop my own research projects, and cemented the reality that there is so much more that we don't know about how the human body works. This community now spans the world and connects thousands of practitioners to researchers—a connection that is vital to future research. The latest insights were presented at the Fifth International Fascia Research Congress in Berlin, Germany, in November 2018. Since my first book was published, research has continued to move ahead in leaps and bounds. Pioneering discoveries have furthered our understanding of the important roles fascia plays in supporting our mobility and overall health. One of the most significant recent findings is Carla Stecco's discovery of a new type of cell in fascia she calls fasciacytes, which may win her the Nobel Prize. This cell specifically produces hyaluronan, a key component facilitating smooth gliding between fascia and muscle. It also promotes the functions of the deep fascia. Stop and think about that: Scientists are finding cells they never knew existed in the human body before now. Imagine how much more there is still to discover.

Not only does fascia play a role supporting our biomechanics, but it plays a significant role in the function of our immune system. The lymphatic system is the most important part of our immune function and overall health, and as it turns out there is no separation between fascia and lymph. The lymphatic system pulls excess fluid and waste proteins from the ECM and interstitial spaces to the pre-lymphatic channels and ultimately out of the body. It also helps with the absorption and transportation of free fatty acids from the digestive system. When flow from the ECM to the lymph is impeded, it causes a wide array of unwanted symptoms. With more research directed to the importance of the interstitial spaces and the fluid flow within, we are gaining new insights on connective tissue functions, elasticity, cancer metastasis, fibrosis, and, of course, the implications of self-care and hands-on therapeutic treatments.

Professor Peter Friedl, MD, PhD, and chair of microscopic cell imaging at Radboud University, and Neil Thiese, MD, professor in the department of pathology at NYU School of Medicine and a leading stem cell researcher, shared their pioneering research on how the mechanisms of disease change the tissues in the human body and how this knowledge can enhance our understanding of cancer and immunotherapies. The pre-lymphatics—what Dr. Friedl called the "conduit" interlinking these systems—are now more understood because of modern microscopy techniques, such as the use of confocal lasers that allow us to visualize living tissue function in a three-dimensional way. Their contributions are helping us better understand how the lymphatic system functions and interlinks to the other tissue structures, including fascia, as well as opening up vital new paths of research about how fascia relates to disease states, fibrosis, and pain.

These preliminary findings, particularly those related to lymph, further validate the importance of fluid flow dynamics, and therefore hydration, for proper stability and overall health.

The primary cells of our connective tissue, called fibroblasts, ensure that the collagen network remains relatively constant in its structure and that the connective tissue maintains its physical characteristics. Like a good housekeeper, they are always scanning the collagen fibrils, fixing and tinkering with them to sustain continuity and integrity. Fibroblasts maintain the interstitial structures that shape the body. This structural homeostasis is critical to the transportation of fluids from the collagen network to the lymphatic system. Both play a significant role in our overall immunity.

▶ Linking the Fascial System to Autonomic Function and Dysfunction

Being sedentary, as well as being overactive, can cause unwanted adaptations to the structural integrity of our fascial system. It's widely understood in the therapeutic community that fascial dysfunction and pain symptoms are inherently linked. We also know movement, muscle contraction, and of course MELT supports fluid mobilization and transportation and can reduce pain symptoms. What I'm proposing is that MELT does far more than just help fascia's supportive qualities: It also aids the regulation of the autonomic functions of the body. Through our clinical research we've shown immediate improvements in heart rate variability and blood pressure recovery using MELT. This is why I call MELT a neurofascial technique. Let me explain how I link fascial dysfunction to altered neurological function including changes in metabolism and hormone balance.

As you learned in Chapter 1, our fascia is a biotensegrity system that gives our body functional structure and provides an environment that enables all body systems to operate in an integrated manner. This pliable collagen system contains many definable components such as adipose tissue, neurovascular sheaths, aponeuroses, epineurium, joint capsules, ligaments, membranes, meninges, retinacula, septa, tendons, visceral fascia, and all the intramuscular and intermuscular connective tissues including endo-/peri-/epimysium.

The superficial fascial layer adheres to the underside of your skin and acts like a sponge. Just like a dried-out sponge, daily living causes this fascial layer, abundant with mechanoreceptors, to become less flexible, adaptable, and resilient. The specific, nuanced use of MELT's soft roller and balls gives our fascia more time to adapt to tension and compression so that we don't overstimulate the billions of sensory nerve endings in this layer. This way, we avoid your brain sending you a pain (trauma) response.

As earlier fascia research has shown, the act of creating slow, gentle tensional length to myofascia—without going too far—actually causes the fascia to rehydrate itself. As this tissue adapts and we apply the compression techniques like Gliding and Shearing, the deeper layers are also affected.

When gliding between fascia layers is impaired, densification and dehydration can occur and affect our range of motion—often causing the sensory receptors to report problems—and can also compromise communication between fibers and cells. Fibrosis, scars, or excessive collagen deposition and cross-linking leads to unwanted connective tissue stiffening as well. This alteration can generate a sense of stiffness and pain, reduce our ability to coordinate movements, cause strain in muscles, create compression in joints, and cause a disconnect in sensorimotor communication. In contrast, resilient fascia (like a moist sponge) is buoyant and adaptable so you can move, stretch, twist, and bend, and consistently return to an ideal, aligned posture.

The science of connective tissue is constantly evolving and expanding, and I can't wait to read about the latest discoveries. If the "why" of this is interesting to you too, I've included a long list of recommended reading at the back of this book.

▶ The Four Rs of MELT: Reconnect, Rebalance, Rehydrate, and Release

Each of the Four Rs of the MELT Method has its own unique techniques that will give you specific results. You'll see some of the elements of the Living Body Model used to simplify what, how, and why you do each R of MELT.

The First R: Reconnect

The first step is learning how to assess where stuck stress is living in your body. To do this, you'll use your Body Sense, not your five common senses. Body Sense is the information taken in and transmitted through the sensory receptors in your connective tissue. This is the foundation of all the Reconnect techniques. It's your body-wide communication system, which you need for efficient movement and balance. Using Body Sense allows you to tune in to where stuck stress is living in your body rather than where you feel pain. You'll learn to identify common imbalances that many of us possess that are left unaddressed from day to day, which is the first step to eliminating them before they cause you pain. I'll review the Rest Assess on page 124 to ensure that you know how to identify these common imbalances using Body Sense.

Reconnect techniques also help recalibrate the part of your nervous system, the Autopilot, that keeps you balanced and stable without thinking about it. One way your Autopilot keeps you balanced is through its connection to your center of gravity, or pelvis. Most of us are out of balance from the effect of stuck stress on our Autopilot. MELT teaches you to identify how the stuck stress in your connective tissue is altering your Autopilot's connection to your center of gravity before this disconnect causes more issues in your overall balance and performance. In the NeuroCore Sequence, I'll teach you a Reconnect move called the Pelvic Tuck and Tilt Challenge to help improve your Autopilot's connection to your center of gravity.

To address the effects of stuck stress—joint compression and instability, imbalance in your core, and faulty sensorimotor control—take a moment to identify your imbalances before treating them with the MELT techniques, then reassess to evaluate the changes. Taking a moment to self-assess your imbalances allows you to identify which areas need your attention and to sense improvements and whole-body changes.

The Rest Assess and Dr. Oz

When *The Melt Method* was published in 2013, I was booked to do a segment on *The Dr. Oz Show*. I saw him when I was about to do a run-through before the taping and asked if I could do a brief MELT sequence with him to show him how quickly I could alter his nervous system and connection with his body. He agreed, and I told him to lie down on the floor. This is what happened:

"Is your mid-back below your shoulder blades on or off the floor?" I asked.

"Off," he replied.

"Are the backs of your thighs on or off the floor?"

"Off."

"In your pelvis, are you feeling more tailbone or butt cheeks?"

"I think my tailbone."

"You just identified three common imbalances. Come up onto the roller," I told him. Once he was lying on the roller, I explained four techniques as he tried them. "So first we're going to reconnect your Autopilot to your center of gravity with two Reconnect moves," I said. "One's called Gentle Rocking, and the other is moving your pelvis without pushing into your feet or moving your ribs." He tried both. "When people have back pain, they can't control or isolate pelvic motion," I added. "This subtle motion I call the Pelvic Tuck and Tilt helps the brain connect to the center of gravity. And then I do a simple technique to stimulate the diaphragmatic motion and then activate the core reflex to rebalance your nervous system and improve your overall balance and stability."

I raced through the techniques with him, and it didn't even take three minutes. Then I told him to get off the roller, lie back down on the floor, and I repeated the three questions.

Assessment is more than a before-and-after comparison—it's a must-do for any sequence as it allows you to evaluate the immediate and specific changes you've made with that particular sequence. You won't have to wonder whether you are doing it right, and you'll learn which moves and sequences lead to the desired results you want to achieve so you save time and effort in the long run. Not only that, but when you reassess and consciously connect with the changes you've made, your Autopilot

"Is your mid-back on or off the floor?" I asked.

"Wow. It's on," he replied.

"Are the backs of your thighs on or off the floor?"

"They're not on the floor, but they're definitely closer."

"In your pelvis, are you feeling more tailbone or butt cheeks?"

"Uh, butt cheeks. That's really interesting."

I smiled. "The cool thing is, doing that helps restore control and balance to your body in just a few minutes. It's the first step in decompressing the unnecessary tension in the low back that often causes low back pain in the first place."

"Who taught you how to do this?" he asked as he sat up.

"I figured this out myself, as a way to simulate what I do with my hands. I call it Hands-Off Bodywork. This way my clients can do it to themselves and not spend so much money and time seeing me in my office."

"Makes sense. I really felt how that changed my back," he said.

"Yes, when people feel the instant changes, they are more likely to do it again. It's what helps them create a self-care practice and stay out of my office," I said as we continued on with the rehearsal.

He truly embraced the power of MELT. During the segment, I also shared microscopic images of fascia in a living body and we tried other MELT techniques with a woman from the audience.

After the show aired, I continued across the country on my first book tour and met thousands of people and shared MELT with them in live events. From teens to elderly adults, some with disabilities and others training for a sport, the participants mentioned the segment as their reason for learning about MELT. It was one of the most inspiring moments in my career—meeting people of all ages and ability levels who came to try MELT for themselves.

resets to a more efficient, balanced state, and its connection with your center of gravity is more precise and integrated. Your nervous system is destressed, and your mind-body communication and connection are heightened. It's as if you actively stepped in and allowed your Autopilot to recalibrate. And another profound result occurs: Your restore regulator gets the opportunity to be dominant while you are awake, so you actually help boost the natural healing mechanisms of your body.

When you do any of the basic MELT sequences, you'll always assess your body for stuck stress, do the sequence, and then reassess to evaluate the changes. Then, once you know how to do the compression or length techniques, you'll add NeuroStrength moves to the sequence to create a MELT Performance Map.

Once you become a savvy MELTer, you'll learn to flip the order of the moves to create new sequences and maps that work toward a desired result. This is another reason why assessing your body first and then reassessing is so important. As you create your own MELT Map, you'll want to know which moves and sequences make the biggest changes. You'll also learn to use moves like the Modified Tuck and Tilt Challenge and Rib Length as movement assessments, which will further enhance your awareness of the profound changes you can make in your own body in just a few minutes a day. In Chapter 11 I'll get you started with maps that have proven to be effective at enhancing sports performance, eliminating joint and muscle pain, and reducing the negative effects of everyday living.

RECONNECT MOVES TO DO:
Rest Assess, Rest Reassess, Pelvic Tuck and Tilt Challenge, Grip Assess, and Autopilot Assessments in MELT Performance Hand and Foot Treatments. Find them on pages 124–141 and 167 in Chapter 5.

The Second R: Rebalance

There are neurological mechanisms that protect our spine and organs while keeping our joints stable and posture aligned. These mechanisms can't be rebalanced through traditional core exercise because they operate without our thinking about them. Stuck stress from our daily life is what causes imbalance in the mechanisms, and it leads to chronic symptoms such as low back pain, lower belly paunch, gut issues, and even weight gain.

To simplify the neurological reflexes and mechanisms that create stability and control, most specifically pelvic control, I created a simple term—the NeuroCore— short for neurological core system. The NeuroCore is responsible for whole-body stabilization and grounding and for the protection of the vital organs. The reflexes and control of this system function autonomically. Doing abdominal exercises will not enhance the control and timing of this deep, intrinsic system. This is why so many people who have strong muscles and work out all the time can still have an imbalanced NeuroCore; many of them, especially body builders, have chronic neck and low back pain or strain. One thing your Autopilot is always trying to do is keep you balanced and stable by allowing for a clear connection to your center of gravity.

The NeuroCore system keeps your spine stable, protects your vital organs, helps with gut issues, and also keeps your body grounded and stable through neurological mechanisms and reflexes. It is not a traditional muscle system; rather, it's a dual neurofascial stabilizing system that functions well out of our conscious control. This complex system of balance is vital to your overall stability and ease of movement.

In my book *The MELT Method*, I shared the Rebalance Sequence using the original MELT soft roller, which is longer than the MELT Performance roller. The Rebalance Sequence directly affects the diaphragm and reflexive core mechanisms. The sequence is so subtle and simple that people often say it doesn't feel like they are

Use Your Body Sense and Always Stop If You Feel Discomfort or Pain

Whenever you MELT, you don't ever want to cause pain. Too much pressure or tension when performing any of the techniques actually decreases the re-hydration effect and increases stuck stress.

You'll know when you're applying too much pressure too fast if you feel discomfort or an area starts to hurt. It might seem counterintuitive, but think about it: If you are in pain, why would you want to cause *more* pain to get out of it? Traditional foam rolling and using hard balls on the body can often cause pain because you go too deep too fast. Most people just roll on these objects and are told that when they find a sensitive area, they should land on it and press harder until the pain decreases.

No part of MELTing should hurt, just as I would never intentionally cause pain with my hands to one of my clients. The pressure should always be tolerable, so listen to your body and ease back your pressure if you feel pain.

doing anything, yet this sequence is incredibly profound. I'll teach you a key technique of the Rebalance Sequence called the 3-D Breath as you will have to learn to activate the core reflex in some of the Performance Sequences.

Another way to create a rebalancing effect is by treating the hands and feet. As this book is geared to those of us looking to improve function and control, I've added the Performance Hand and Foot Treatments to work directly on the Rooted Core mechanisms on pages 129–141. These specific techniques help improve grip, balance, and overall functional integrity and also cause a rebalancing effect.

Treating your feet helps ground reaction, timing, and control when you move and also reduces low back compression. It doesn't matter whether you play a sport or you just want to walk with ease—foot treatments are a must for anyone. Treating your hands helps with grip and releases unnecessary tension in your forearms, shoulders, and neck. Who doesn't want their hands to work better? With all the time we spend trying to make our butts look lifted in our jeans, we should spend an equal amount of time treating our hands and feet. As you age, I'm telling you, you won't care about how lifted your butt looks in your pants—but you *will* care if you can't lift your butt up from a chair without a struggle! You can do these quick treatments anywhere, and they take only about five minutes, so let's try them both.

REBALANCE MOVES TO DO:
The MELT Performance Hand and Foot Treatments with soft and firm balls.
Find them on pages 129–141 in Chapter 5.

Finding Your Core Reflex Using the 3-D Breath

When we think of the core, we think of crunches and achieving flat abs. Deeper than the superficial muscles that give the appearance of a six-pack, there are muscles that stabilize the spine and keep your organs supported and protected. Even if you exercise, the function of this deeper, neurological core system can be faulty. It's inherently linked to your diaphragm and you can improve and restore its function if you know how. You can do this with a technique I call a focused breath. Let's see whether you can sense what it feels like when you consciously connect to your core reflex:

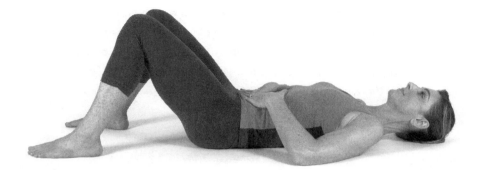

▶ *Lie on your back with your knees bent and feet on the floor.*

▶ *Place both hands on your belly. Think of your torso like an egg-shaped cylinder. Take a focused, slightly slower breath than normal into your entire torso. Imagine expanding an egg's center yolk to the shell of the egg. Sense with your hands how your belly expands three-dimensionally on the inhale. As you exhale, sense how your belly deflates three-dimensionally back to the center of the yolk. During natural exhalation, the core reflex involuntarily activates, it's just subtle so we don't necessarily feel it. Take another focused inhale but this time to consciously activate your core reflex, force your exhale out by creating a* shhh *sound (like you would to keep someone quiet). The increased pressure you create can enhance your sense of the core reflex—a cylindrical, three-dimensional inward gathering type contraction, more subtle and soft than doing an abdominal crunch. It's a deep sensation, not superficial.*

▶ *Try this forced exhale again but try making a* ssss *sound (like a deflating tire) to heighten your ability to sense the reflexive action in your deep abdomen. Then try a* haaa *sound (like fogging up a mirror). Which sound gives you enhanced awareness of the cylindrical contraction that subtly squeezes your spine, pelvic floor, and organs from all sides as you force the exhale?*

▶ *Pick the sound that best allows you to sense this inward contraction or hugging sensation in your belly and try it one more time.*

▶ *Now take a natural inhale and on your exhale, without forcing your exhale with a sound, allow your natural exhale to come out of your body and in the middle of your exhale, see if you can consciously connect to your core reflex and enhance your sense of that contraction.*

If a natural breathing pattern exists, the belly and chest expand outward on your inhale, and on your exhale, the cylinder of the torso contracts inward. Emotional stress, pain, and daily repetitive habits can alter this natural motion of the diaphragm and contraction of the core reflex.

If you can sense this rhythmical motion of a relaxed belly expansion on your

The Importance of Breathing During NeuroStrength

We take breathing for granted, partly because we don't have to think about it. We inhale and exhale twenty-eight thousand times a day (give or take). However, everything from emotional trauma to daily stress, pregnancy, injury, and even just habitual movements and postures can alter natural and rhythmic breathing patterns.

Ideally, when we inhale, the belly and torso expand outward; and on a natural exhale, the belly and torso move inward toward our midline or center. However, many people, when they take a breath in, find that their belly moves inward and their shoulders shrug and move upward; and as they exhale, their belly paunches outward. This is called a faulty breathing pattern, or what I call reversed breathing mechanics. Often, I have clients who inhale deeply, barely exhale, and then quickly breathe in again. Others have a shallow inhale but seem to exhale for days.

Restoring proper diaphragmatic motion and the activation of our natural core reflex was an integral part of the Rebalance Sequence in the MELT Method book. With MELT Performance, you will prepare for reintegration by "finding your core."

When you're doing MELT Performance, the opportunity to find your core by slowing down and slightly forcing your exhale with the *shhh*, *ssss*, or *haaa* sound helps engage the core reflex. Ideally, over time you can feel and follow your exhale and consciously connect to the core reflex without forcing the exhale or making any sound. It's the easiest way to rebalance the stress and

inhale and connect to the inward gathering of your core reflex on your exhale, you're
retraining and strengthening your core far beyond any abdominal exercise.

Consciously connecting to this contraction is what I call finding your core. Later,
when we try the NeuroCore Stability Sequence (Chapter 8), this will be an important
factor in executing the techniques to improve core stabilization and control.

restore regulator. Although many involuntary and autonomic functions occur from day to day, the one that's easiest for us to access and control is breathing. You can't think your way to digesting food faster or having an epic bowel movement when you're constipated. But you certainly can think about taking a breath in and consciously connecting to the core reflex and sensing its three-dimensional engagement. In doing so, you are truly improving natural and autonomic regulation by doing very little.

This is also one of the reasons why breathing techniques are so soothing during stressful moments, because you're quieting the stress reflex, boosting repair, and rewriting your neurological pathways back to normal functioning. If you want to create neurological regulation, the easiest no-brainer way to do so is through the diaphragm.

Your diaphragm is your body's breathing apparatus, the primary oscillator that the brain signals to contract so many times throughout the day. Imagine if you had to tell yourself to breathe 24/7. You'd find yourself gasping for air, and you'd never get anything done because you'd be worried about passing out from a lack of oxygen.

But when you think about it, people stop breathing properly all the time. Have you ever been sitting at your desk reading, and then all of a sudden you find yourself inhaling really deeply? You didn't consciously do that. Your brain did it for you, because it realized it needed more oxygen and you needed to expand your diaphragm more.

Before you execute any of the NeuroStrength moves, I'll invite you to find your core to set your body up for restoring optimal stability and function. Much like the setup, tuning back in to and focusing on your core between repetitions is a great practice to refine your ability to restore stability.

▶ The Long-Reaching Effects of Abdominal Surgery and Scarring

Your skin is connected on a neurological level to your entire body and to all its systems, including emotions. It sends and receives information to and from the brain through neurons and receptors. When you get a cut on your skin, your brain sends a message and you react—and so does your body.

Abdominal or visceral surgery—a C-section or removal of the appendix or gallbladder, for example—can alter NeuroCore communication. NeuroCore, as you know, is my simplified term for the inherent connections between the brain, the viscera (your organs), and your center of gravity (your pelvis). Surgery that cuts into all of the layers of a body means that something that is usually in constant communication is disrupted. Collagen fibrils are severed, and after closure and repair of the initial cut, the scar tissue that develops can cause significant alterations on many levels—structural, emotional, and neurological. Adhesions after visceral surgery are very common but are often undetected until pain in the low back or pelvic floor or issues such as incontinence, bowel distress, or prolapse arise. These issues can take years to develop, and the link to the abdominal surgery is often disregarded.

In addition, no matter how small or perfect a scar looks on the skin's surface, the collagen network attached to its underside is forever changed. A C-section cuts and alters every fascial layer, no matter how exquisite a surgeon's skills. And if the C-section was the result of an emergency, the stress and trauma of that event is stored not just in the mother's mind, but in her tissues as well. Furthermore, cutting into these layers abundant with sensory nerves also affects the nervous system. Many women are left feeling numb in their abdomen, even far away from the scar. I've worked on hundreds of women who come to me because of low back pain, and they have no idea that the obvious culprit is their C-section scar—especially if they gave birth years before.

Scar tissue from any abdominal surgery can cause instability and dysfunction in your neurofascial components. But no matter how long you have had a scar, take heart, as you can help reduce unnecessary adhesions and restore both fascial and neurological stability. One of the many benefits of the NeuroCore Stability Sequence is that you can finally feel your tissue again while decreasing pain in your low back and numbness in your pelvis.

Scar Tissue and Your Core

I've coined the terms *Reflexive Core* and *Rooted Core* to describe the dual neurofascial stabilizing system. The neurological core system has little to nothing to do with the strength of your abdominal muscles. I want you to forget all about muscles— what's important to stability is how your nervous system and connective tissues sustain connection from your brain to your body and body to brain.

The *Reflexive Core* has a primary job of supporting, protecting, and stabilizing the gut-to-brain communication and the structures within its walls. This aspect of your core, on a physiological level, consists of billions of neurons, efferent and afferent sensory nerves, and fascial receptors that monitor, adapt, and respond to everything we do. It's always on and is described as a tonic system (constant low load contraction). It never rests. It's not a phasic muscle system like your rectus abdominis (aka your six pack), whose primary job is to contract when you move your torso into flexion.

Any kind of abdominal surgery can alter the natural, neurological reflexive nature of this system ultimately leading to overactivation of superficial muscles like rectus abdominis and external obliques.

The *Rooted Core* also has a primary job—to sustain the fine balance of the masses and spaces to ensure that our innate joint congruity stays in an adequate range. It has both fascial and neurological connectivity from head to toe and manages to balance us when we stand, walk, or otherwise move. When we rest, lie down, and give in to gravity, its level of activation ideally changes.

Through fascia, these systems are connected to the diaphragm, which is a doorway to restoring NeuroCore function and connection.

The NeuroCore Stability Sequence shows you how to access the core reflex. It will help you enhance or restore the Reflexive Core and restore the rooting or grounding mechanisms of the Rooted Core. Even if you have scars from a long-ago abdominal surgery, being able to restore function on the NeuroStrength level goes far beyond muscle strength.

The Third R: Rehydrate

Restoring the fluid state of your connective tissue is at the heart of the MELT Method and MELT Performance. It's as important to your health as a balanced diet, restful sleep, and regular activity. Beyond chronic pain, dehydrated connective tissue can cause many seemingly unrelated common symptoms like headaches, low-grade inflammation, and muscle weakness. Even wrinkles and cellulite are caused by connective tissue issues.

The Rehydrate techniques are directed to the health of the connective tissue system. Interestingly, tension and compression—the very things that cause dehydration in the first place—can also help rehydrate your connective tissue once you know how to do it.

When your connective tissue is properly hydrated, your muscles work better, your joints have the support and space they need, and your body is better aligned to help absorb the physical shocks and emotional stresses of daily living. By restoring the tissue that supports your joints, your overall neurological reception is enhanced, which makes you better prepared to restore joint stability and control with the reintegration techniques.

The MELT Rehydrate techniques include three types of positive compression—Gliding, Shearing, and Rinsing—and Two-Directional Length techniques to stimulate the different receptors, cells, collagen fibrils, and fluids of the connective tissue. These techniques create a rehydration effect similar to hands-on therapy.

Rehydrate is done with MELT's soft roller and small hand and foot treatment balls. For the MELT compression techniques, the soft roller provides gentle, positive compression for the part of your body that is on the roller without overstimulating or stressing the connective tissue and nervous system. For MELT length techniques, the MELT soft roller stabilizes, elevates, and gently supports your spine, ribs, or pelvis so you can find the proper position to acquire adequate tensional pull in specific regions of the body. These techniques can create whole-body changes in just minutes. Remember, you always want to maintain tolerable pressure during any of the compression techniques. Pain is your signal that the compression is too much.

Positive Compression Techniques

Gliding

When I work with my hands on a client, I can easily adjust the amount of pressure I apply to acquire the changes that need to be made. If you use a firm, stiff object to treat your tissues, on the other hand, you have a greater chance of going too deep, too fast, causing pain but not necessarily creating positive changes in the tissue. Developing a soft roller was necessary so my clients could gain the same results as with my hands-on treatment.

Gliding is a two-directional preparatory technique, designed to give the sensory receptors in the superficial fascia and the tissue itself time to adapt to compression. This small back-and-forth motion also acts as an exploratory technique to help you investigate and identify areas where the tissue has lost some of its adaptability.

As you Glide, you may notice areas that are sensitive and tender or feel restricted, stiff, or lumpy. These barriers are what you want to learn to identify. The sensitivity you feel is your body's way of letting you know that these areas need some help. Once you learn to find these barriers, you'll edge up against them—what I call meeting the barrier—rather than compressing them directly to prepare for a Shearing technique.

Shearing

When I find a barrier during a hands-on treatment, I do a common therapeutic technique called shearing. To develop a hands-off self-treatment, I experimented with a variety of pressures and durations to create positive changes without inflicting pain. With the soft roller, I found I could mimic shearing using two types of compression techniques, which I call Direct Shearing and Indirect Shearing.

When you find a barrier, you'll edge up against it rather than landing on the center of it to create the Shear. Shearing stimulates the cells, fibers, and receptors living in your fascia. After creating a Shear, you'll wait for a moment to induce what's called the piezoelectric effect. When you release the compression, fascia generates an electric charge in response to the applied mechanical stress and shear. This is the first step in enhancing connective tissue's elastic and supportive qualities.

Regardless of which type of Shear you do, the roller is not moving against your skin. Instead, you're using this tool to compress and "pin" the skin so you can cause a type of friction between the underlying tissues.

Of all the MELTing techniques, Shearing is the most intense, but you want to make sure you aren't inflicting so much pressure that you feel pain. When you Shear, you are in control of how much pressure you apply, but if the tissue has lost its elastic qualities, some areas will be sensitive. The more relaxed you keep your muscles while you Shear, the more effective your self-treatment will be.

> DIRECT SHEARING: While sustaining consistent pressure on the roller with a body part, you'll create a twisting or kneading movement. Think of using your bone like you would the heel of your hand to knead dough. The roller is stationary when you do this. Direct Shearing allows you to mobilize and rehydrate the tissue from skin to bone. The smaller the region you Shear, the better the rehydration effect.

INDIRECT SHEARING: This technique uses muscle contraction to shear the tissues between the skin and bones. If you sustain consistent pressure with your body weight on the roller and move a nearby joint, you'll contract and release the muscles and cause them to move against the compression. This stimulates and hydrates the deep layers of connective tissue that surround your muscles and bones, which helps to restore the gliding movement around your muscles. This is a key factor to restoring proper muscle timing and tone.

Here is an easy way to experience these two types of shear using your hands: Grab and squeeze the middle of your right forearm with your left hand. Now rotate your right forearm left to right. This is a *Direct Shear*. Your flesh isn't rubbing against your left hand; rather, you're creating friction in the layers of tissue between your skin and your forearm bones. To experience an *Indirect Shear*, keep the squeeze on your forearm while you flex and extend your wrist. If you feel the muscles contracting under your grip, you're sensing how you can stimulate the tissue underneath your skin by moving a nearby joint.

Rinsing

The goal of Rinsing is to take the local fluid exchange that Shearing creates and move it globally to affect the entire fascial network. Fascia is a continuous matter so you can affect the entire system without touching every square inch of your body. After a few Rinsing passes, all of the fluid is moving in the same direction in a vortex-like motion. Like moving water in a tub, you don't need to touch all the water within the tub to get it to move.

Rinsing enhances the tensional energy within the fascial system. Both the nervous system and our cells rely on the fluid flow of connective tissue to transport information and nutrients throughout your entire body and move unwanted matter into the lymphatic channels and out of the tissues so new fluids can enter. To get the most out of Rinsing, keep your pressure consistent and move swiftly in the right direction.

POSITIVE COMPRESSION REHYDRATE TECHNIQUES TO DO:
Upper Body Rehydrate Sequence, Seated Compression Sequence,
Lower Body Rehydrate Sequence, Neck Release Sequence,
MELT Performance Hand and Foot Treatments, and SI Joint Shear.
Find them on pages 129–180 in Chapter 5.

Two-Directional Length Techniques

Unlike traditional muscle stretching, MELT's Two-Directional Length techniques are designed to cause a subtle tensional pull in the fascia to restore its elastic and supportive qualities. The tension you create pulls fluid out of the connective tissue, and when you let the tension go, fluid returns to the microvacuolar spaces. Much like Rinsing, releasing the tension initiates a powerful global fluid exchange, which can create changes you'll be able to sense when you reassess.

Two-Directional Length involves using muscles to move specific masses of the body away from each other in equal timing. For example, when you do Hip to Heel Press, you have to tilt your pelvis and flex your heel at the same time with the same amount of effort in opposing directions. If your knee bends as you do this, you lose the full effect of the tensional pull from hip to heel. Focus on sensing a cohesive fascial pull from end to end rather than trying to feel your muscles stretch. (Think of pulling on a rubber band in two directions.) Once you have the proper position and tension, you'll hold it for two or three focused breaths at most.

To get full contact with the tissue, you must use specific muscles to correctly align your joints. Engaging your core muscles will help you gain stability and maintain the proper position.

TWO-DIRECTIONAL LENGTH TECHNIQUES TO DO:
Hip to Heel Press, Figure 4, Bent Knee Press, and Rib Length.
Find them on pages 145–166 in Chapter 5.

The Fourth R: Release

Daily aches, tension, and stiffness in the neck, low back, hands, and feet are so common that even athletes and young people think they're normal. These are the areas that bear the greatest burden from stuck stress.

I've never heard anyone complain about getting taller as they get older. We just seem to lose space in our joints and expect to shrink as we age. When the bones of your spine move closer to each other, the discs in between your vertebrae and the nerves that radiate out from your spinal column also become compressed. This causes pain. And any pain caused by compression is a sign that you have inflammation in your connective tissue, which can lead to joint damage. Sensory and motor communication can become impaired and delayed, leading to a more misaligned spine. Your Autopilot must then work a lot harder just to maintain a misaligned posture.

Losing joint space is less about aging and more about daily repetition and unaddressed stuck stress in your connective tissue. That's why twisting your low back and cracking your knuckles or your neck never seem to help because these moves don't address the cause of the pain. And by the way, doing such things can actually increase damaging stress and compression.

When you do the Release techniques, you'll use small, focused movements to bring fluid flow back to the vital spaces of the neck, low back, hands, feet, and other joints that are challenged to remain stable from overuse, disuse, and accumulated

The Indirect Before Direct Approach

A key concept in MELT is the Indirect Before Direct approach. Every good manual therapist should treat you that way!

The Indirect Before Direct concept is this: If you tell me you have pain in your neck, I find all the other problems, test and retest, work on the hidden culprits, before I go close to where you tell me the pain is. I want to work on your hands, upper back, and even your legs before I add a neck-release move. I know when your neck hurts that you want to rub and dig into it—but trust me, your neck is the victim. If someone was crying out for your help you wouldn't beat them up to stop their crying. Don't beat your body up to make it stop hurting. Our first objective is to improve the sliding and gliding movement in your connective tissue so your body moves more efficiently.

Another benefit of the Indirect Before Direct approach is that if you have pain in a certain location, the more you focus on it, the worse it's going to feel. You're going to tell yourself that you can't get better until somebody helps you with that specific pain—and that thought virus can get lodged and take its toll. When treatment is shifted away from the painful area, however, the thought virus can be neutralized, and healing can be a much speedier process.

stuck stress. You'll also decompress unnecessary tension in the vital spaces that become misaligned and restricted from daily living.

These powerful techniques release joint compression and relieve tension and pain. The result is better range of motion and improved posture. And remember: Before you release your neck or low back, always rehydrate your tissue first. This is how you will achieve the greatest result in the least amount of time.

RELEASE TECHNIQUE TO DO:

Neck Release Sequence. Find it on pages 176–180 in Chapter 5.

▶ Tips to Make MELT Performance Work for You

There are three foundational Rehydrate sequences for MELT Performance— Upper Body Rehydrate Sequence, Lower Body Rehydrate Sequence, and Seated Compression Sequence. I've added the Low Back Decompress move to your Lower Body Rehydrate Sequence, as well as a Neck Release Sequence, because who doesn't need a little relief in their neck and low back? You can mix and match these sequences, or use just some of the moves to create a unique MELT Map.

Here are some tips for making MELT Performance work for you:

- Combining multiple sequences creates a MELT Map. This can make your MELTing take a little bit longer, but you'll have much more profound results.

- MELT techniques help improve the fluid and nutrient absorption of every cell in your body. So to get immediate and lasting results, drink water before and after you MELT.

- All the MELT compression techniques are done only on your body's masses, like the upper back, hips, and thighs. We *never* compress the spaces, like the neck, low back, or behind the knees. These spaces will benefit from work done above and below them rather than directly on them.

- The more often you MELT, the fewer barriers you will find. Some areas of the body, such as near the deep or side hip, especially closer to the joints, have more dense, fibrous layers of connective tissue. These regions of the body are frequently strained by our repetitive postures and hold more barriers, causing muscles to become inhibited; you'll notice this when you MELT these areas, as they can be extremely tender. If this happens, it's your cue to ease off pressure in order to achieve the most beneficial results.

- Remember, you want to "wake up a little something" in your connective tissue, not overstimulate it or the sensory nervous system. Overstimulation can create inflammation and reduce the benefits of your self-treatment—and MELT is designed to reduce pain and inflammation, not increase it. Your connective tissue responds to a specific amount of pressure applied in a precise manner. Applying too much pressure, moving too fast, and staying on an area too long actually decrease the benefits of MELT.

- Last but never least—and I can't emphasize this enough!—in order to get the full benefits of MELT, it is important to listen to your body and make adjustments when (or ideally before) you feel pain. When you experience an intense sensation, pull back the amount of pressure you are applying and Glide more if needed.

In Chapter 6, you'll learn about the Two Rs of NeuroStrength: Reintegrate and Repattern. Because the neurological pathways that dictate motor control must be clear and open, you will always incorporate at least Reconnect and Rehydrate at the beginning of each sequence; and for some sequences, you'll do all Four Rs in addition to Reintegrate and Repattern. Your body will *always* respond better to any MELT Performance moves when your connective tissue is properly hydrated, so practice these basic techniques and sequences if you are new to MELT so your body is ready to reintegrate stability.

5

MELT Rehydrate and Release Sequences

Preparing your body for improved stability and motor control is essential to gaining fast, long-lasting results. The Four Rs of MELT give your body an added boost of both awareness and stability that no exercise or dietary program can achieve.

Before you jump into the NeuroStrength moves, make sure you are savvy with the Rest Assess and using your Body Sense. This way, you can tune into your current imbalances and quickly learn which moves give you instant results. Also, adding the Performance Hand and Foot Treatments to your practice every day is one of the easiest ways to rebalance your NeuroCore, which is why they come first in this chapter. They are also quick treatments that give your grip and balance an added boost.

In fact, for those of us who play a sport or engage in any fitness-related activity or exercise program, both of these treatments will give you a competitive edge. MELTing your hands and feet can help with hand-eye coordination, speed, and agility. You can do these treatments on their own or add them to a roller sequence for greater results.

Remember, if you currently have an injury or pain, the Hand and Foot Treatments can become the indirect approach to help you reduce unnecessary inflammation and restore control. Before you begin the Upper Body Stability moves, doing the Upper Body Rehydrate Sequence will help you reintegrate the timing of the deep stabilizing mechanisms of your shoulder girdle and shoulder joint. Adequate tone in your connective tissue leads to improved supportive qualities before you move. Your motor timing will become more accurate, and you will Reintegrate more quickly if you Rehydrate first.

Finally, releasing unnecessary tension in your neck or low back is a great thing for anyone to learn to do! If you find that your neck gets tight when you do the Upper Body Stability Sequence—even if you started with the Upper Body Rehydrate Sequence—add the Neck Release before you try it the next time. For so many of us, our daily life leads to excessive tension and compression in these two primary spaces of the body. I do the Neck Release Sequence every night before I go to bed because it helps me get to sleep faster and sleep more soundly. It's a fast treatment, and much like the MELT Performance Hand Treatment, it can offer indirect changes through your entire body.

This chapter presents the following MELT moves in different sequences:

Reconnect

Rest Assess and Rest Reassess

Modified Tuck and Tilt Challenge

Pelvic Tuck and Tilt Challenge

Neck Turn Assess and Reassess

Rebalance

Performance Hand Treatment

Mini Performance Hand Treatment

Performance Foot Treatment

Mini Performance Foot Treatment

3-D Breath

Rehydrate: Compression

Upper Back Glide and Shear

Inner Shoulder Blade Glide and Shear

Side Rib Glide and Outer Shoulder Blade Glide and Shear

❯ Rest Assess and Rest Reassess

The Rest Assess

Before you start any MELT sequence, you need to identify stuck stress and how it's affecting your body. Practice the Rest Assess now before we jump into the other techniques.

Stuck stress displaces the ideal placement of your masses and spaces—I call the areas on the floor masses and the areas off the floor spaces—as it accumulates in three regions: the shoulder girdle, diaphragm, and pelvis.

❯ *Lie on your back with your palms face up and your arms and legs extended. Take a breath into your body and begin to notice that some areas of your body are naturally touching the floor and some areas are lifted off the floor. If you can notice this without moving, touching, or looking at your body, you are already using Body Sense.*

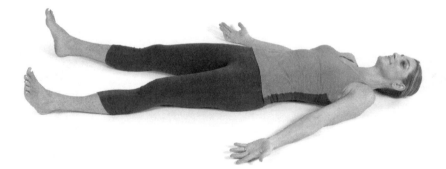

❯ **SHOULDER GIRDLE:** *If stuck stress accumulates in the shoulder girdle, it will displace all of the upper body masses from their ideal positions. If it's left unaddressed, your chances of developing shoulder, neck, elbow, and wrist pain are increased.*

   – IDEAL: *Head is weighted right behind the bridge of your nose, arms are evenly balanced from left to right, and the torso weight is sensed in the mid-rib wall, where women define the bra line, just below the shoulder blades.*

- WHAT YOU MIGHT FEEL: *Head feels off-center, one arm feels more weighted, or all of your back weight feels like it's propped on your shoulder blades.*

- *If you're not sure what you feel using Body Sense, slowly turn your head left and right to notice whether stuck stress is causing issues in your neck. Sensing pain in your neck or limited range of motion to either side, or noticing that your shoulder lifts as you turn your head away from it are signs of stuck stress as well.*

▶ **DIAPHRAGM:** *If stuck stress lives in the diaphragm, it will change the shape and size of your low back curve and inhibit your ability to take a full breath.*

- IDEAL: *The curve of your low back is a small, distinctive space below the belly button. When you inhale, your belly and rib region expand evenly and effortlessly on all sides.*

- WHAT YOU MIGHT FEEL: *The arch of your low back curve feels more like a mid-back curve, with the highest point of the curve above the navel. When you inhale, your breath may feel limited to just your chest or restricted.*

- *If you're not sure what you feel using Body Sense, use the common sense of touch. Rather than touch your low back, put one of your fingers in your belly button. Notice whether the curve of your low back feels like a small, distinctive space from the belly button to the pelvis or whether the highest point of the curve is above the navel.*

▶ **PELVIS:** *If stuck stress accumulates in the pelvis, it will displace all of the lower body masses and spaces.*

- IDEAL: *The mass of your pelvis feels evenly weighted on both butt cheeks, the backs of your thighs and calves feel evenly weighted, your knee and ankle spaces feel evenly lifted from the floor, and your feet are evenly angled outward like a letter V.*

- WHAT YOU MIGHT FEEL: *Your sacrum or tailbone are on the floor, the backs of the thighs or calves feel unevenly weighted or entirely off the floor on one or both sides, your knee and ankle spaces are unevenly lifted, or your feet feel turned way out to the sides of the room, pointed away from your ankles, or at completely different angles.*

▶ *This may seem like a lot of things to remember, but the more you practice this Rest Assess the easier it will be to identify imbalances caused by stuck stress. Of all the imbalances you might feel, I want you to tune in to four in particular as these are the ones that compress the neck and low back unnecessarily and destabilize the NeuroCore.*

▶ *When you lie on the floor, whether it's before you MELT or go for a run, play ball, do yoga, or just go to work, if you feel like*

    1. all of your back weight is propped on your shoulder blades,

    2. your mid-back is arched off the floor,

    3. your tailbone is more weighted than your butt cheeks, or

    4. the backs of your thighs are off the floor,

you should spend at least ten minutes a day trying to eliminate these imbalances so they don't accumulate and cause more issues.

▶ *I also want you to learn to identify whether this accumulated stress is altering your Autopilot's connection to your center of gravity and ultimately its efficiency in keeping you stable.*

▶ *Lying on your back, sense the entire left and right sides of your body. Do you feel balanced from left to right—or does one side of your body feel heavier or one leg feel longer?*

▶ *Remember, one of the functions of the Autopilot is to regulate your body's balance and stability during movement and rest. If you sense that one entire side of your body feels more weighted to the floor or one leg feels longer than the other, this is your sign that your Autopilot has lost its clear connection to your body's center of gravity. As a result, your Autopilot has to work harder to keep you balanced from day to day—even when you're at rest. This is a key reason people feel exhausted or agitated even when they try to rest.*

If it's your first time using Body Sense and you're not sure what you feel, that's okay. Don't get frustrated. Learning to use Body Sense to identify common imbalances takes practice. Once we do some of the techniques and reassess, you might notice that something feels different. Each time you MELT, do a Rest Assess first and you

Signs of Stuck Stress

	What's Ideal	What Common Imbalances You Might Feel When Stuck Stress Accumulates
Shoulder Girdle	Head centered	Head off-center
	Arms evenly weighted	One arm more weighted
	Mid-ribs weighted below shoulder blades where women define the bra line	Most weight on shoulder blades, mid-ribs feel lifted away from the floor
	Head turns evenly left to right	Limited range of motion to one side or pain
Diaphragm	Small distinctive space in the low back, with the highest point of the curve sensed below the navel	Mid-back arch from your pelvis to your shoulder blades, highest point of the curve above the navel
Pelvic Girdle	Evenly weighted buttocks	Weight on tailbone or buttocks unevenly weighted
	Back of thighs on the ground evenly	Back of thighs off the ground or unevenly weighted
	Knee space evenly off the ground	Knee space uneven or unnoticeable
	Calves evenly weighted	One calf more weighted
	Ankle space evenly lifted	Outer ankle bones touch the floor
	Outer heel weighted, toes angle where ceiling meets the wall	Toes point to sides of the room or down and away from ankle bones or at different angles
Autopilot	Left and right sides of your body feel balanced	One side of the body feels more weighted or one leg feels longer

will develop your ability to use Body Sense, which is the first and most important part of self-care. Learning to identify and deal with the possible culprits behind pain rather than focusing on pain symptoms can in fact decrease your sense of pain in the first place!

Once you understand the signs of stuck stress you are trying to identify, it will become easier for you to assess, taking you two minutes or less.

Remember: It doesn't matter how good you get at doing the MELT techniques; if you don't assess before and then reassess after, you are missing the most critical part of the protocol and reducing your Autopilot's ability to reset.

Rest Reassess

After you do any sequence, you'll return to the Rest Assess position to reassess and evaluate the changes the sequence makes. You may find that treating your upper body makes noticeable changes in your lower body and vice versa. This is important to notice as you create your own MELT Map.

It's not uncommon for people to have low back or hip pain because their torso is full of stuck stress, limiting their pelvic stability and leg control. When you return to the Rest Reassess, notice if you've eliminated any of the common imbalances.

In your upper body, ideally your head and arms feel more centered and balanced, and you notice more rib weight instead of being propped up on your shoulder blades. You may also be able to turn your head more easily from left to right.

You may also notice the shape and size of your low back is less arched, and your lower body masses and spaces may also feel more ideally placed.

One of the most profound sensations to feel is the Autopilot reconnecting to your center of gravity. Often, after doing a full MELT Map my clients will say they don't feel their left and right sides anymore and instead they feel the wave formation of the masses and spaces flowing on and off the floor from head to toe.

Remember, reassessing not only allows you to identify whether your self-care has had an effect, it allows your Autopilot to reset and acquire better neurological connection to your center of gravity. Allow these changes to set into your body for a moment before doing another sequence or going about your day.

❱ MELT Performance Hand and Foot Treatments

To improve sports performance we train and practice drills. However, the two most used parts of our body, our hands and feet, get little to no attention—no matter what kind of lifestyle we lead. Carpal tunnel syndrome, weak grip, neuromas, plantar fasciitis, and other hand and foot issues can end a sports career, not to mention hinder daily activities. The Hand and Foot Treatments use all Four Rs, create global effects to the neurofascial system, and are safe to do every day. Doing either before you train can give your entire body better grounding and overall coordination.

Rather than doing the Rest Assess, you'll use the Grip Assess to evaluate whether stuck stress is inhibiting the strength of your grip, and a standing Body Scan Assess to determine whether your Autopilot is functioning efficiently and has a clear connection to your center of gravity. Both treatments help rebalance the Autopilot because billions of sensory nerve endings live in our hands and feet. Stimulating them can create body-wide signaling and help your Autopilot's GPS-like tracking system by releasing tension in the many joints of your hands and feet.

The other great thing about the Hand and Foot Treatments is that you learn the basic compression techniques of MELT. The Glide, Shear, and Rinse process improves the overall supportive qualities of your fascia.

Just like using the Rest Assess, you will learn how to assess your hand grip and test your Autopilot's efficiency in a standing posture. Here are a few things to bear in mind:

- No matter how good you become at doing these treatments, make sure you assess before you treat and reassess right after to sense any changes your self-care practice has achieved.

- Once you are competent in the techniques, any Hand or Foot Treatment should take you fewer than ten minutes.

- Gliding is a preparatory technique when you use the large soft ball. Adding the large firm ball to your treatment can add awareness with an investigative touch. If your connective tissue isn't in an ideal state, you can often feel the texture of it while you Glide. If you sense what feels like grains of rice or bumps—or what some of my clients call shards of glass—that's what dehydration feels like. So when you Glide, you aren't going to change the tissue in any profound way;

rather, you are giving it time to subtly adapt and prepare it for the Shear while you build your Body Sense and learn to apply tolerable pressure without pain.

- When you Shear tissue, you are trying to cause two surfaces to shift in opposition to one another. When you properly Shear, you aren't working at the level of the skin but at the level of what's between the underlying skin and superficial fascial layer and your bones. You are creating friction along with compression and moderate force to induce changes in the collagen matrix. Remember, collagen is a conductor. When you Shear, you are changing the tensile stress on the collagen fibrils. This is a key factor in pushing or pumping fluids out of the small spaces between the collagen bindings where the pressure is. Similar to working fluid into a sponge, once fluid adaptation occurs, you compress and wait so when you decompress you get a "fill" effect in the tissue layers. This enhances the sliding and gliding of the collagen fibrils, improving the tissue's supportive qualities. Don't forget that compressing and waiting for a moment after you Shear will result in the greatest changes. Give your tissue a moment to adapt to create a local fluid exchange.

- Once you create local fluid changes in the connective tissue system, you'll Rinse to induce force in a specific direction, making a global fluid exchange throughout the entire tissue matrix. Moving fluid in one direction for a period of time creates both chemical and electrical changes similar to a vortex. This induces cell-to-cell communication as well as stimulating sensory nerve endings. Rinsing can cause many global changes in the neurofascial system, improving stability and mobility.

- You'll also add the Friction technique to stimulate blood flow and circulation as an added bonus. This gently stimulates the lymphatic system and can help reduce low-grade swelling or inflammation in your hands and feet. When you do this technique, you are gently rubbing the ball against your skin with a very light and superficial pressure.

▶ Performance Hand Treatment

You will need a large soft and a large firm ball.

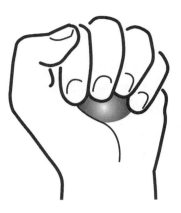

LARGE SOFT BALL

Grip Assess

▶ *Hold a large soft ball in one hand and squeeze 3 or 4 times. Now try it with your other hand. Can you easily create a powerful grip? Does one hand feel stronger than the other? Do you sense tension in either forearm when you create a strong grip?*

Glide

▶ *Place the ball between your hands, interlace your fingers, and rub the ball from point 3 across the base of the palm to point 5 and return to point 3 with equal pressure.*

▶ *Continue Gliding the ball back and forth at the base of your palm for 20 to 30 seconds.*

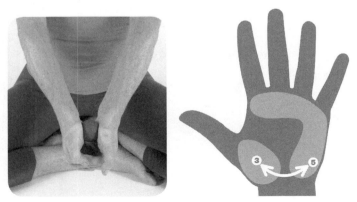

Direct Shear

▶ *Place the ball under point 3, the thumb pad, and create small circles in either direction for approximately 30 seconds. When you are doing this correctly, the ball barely moves.*

▶ *Gently compress the ball between your thumb pads and wait. Hold the compression and take two focused breaths as you allow the tissue to adapt.*

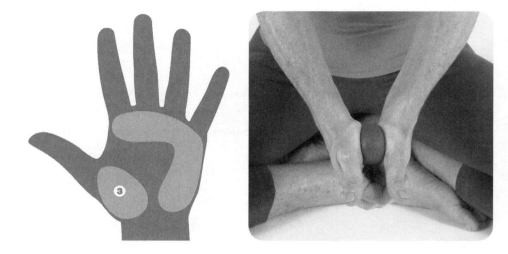

Indirect Shear

▶ *With the ball under point 3, the thumb pad, maintain tolerable pressure while you move the thumbs in and out to indirectly Shear the tissue. Take three or four focused breaths.*

▶ *Hold the compression and take two focused breaths as you allow the tissue to adapt.*

Forearm Rinse

▶ *Starting with the ball under your fingers, slowly press the ball toward your wrist and up your forearm to your elbow in a continuous motion.*

▶ *Repeat the Rinsing motion 8 to 10 times in one direction, from fingers to elbow. Take focused breaths and maintain consistent pressure.*

▶ *Switch hands and repeat.*

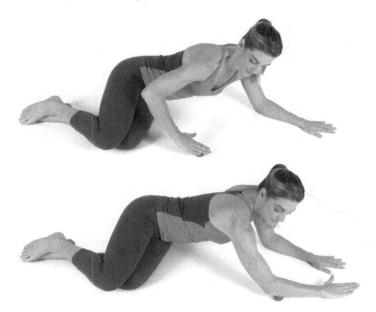

LARGE FIRM BALL

Repeat these techniques—Glide, Direct Shear, Indirect Shear, and Forearm Rinse— with the large firm ball. This ball won't compress like the soft ball so don't press harder. If you find using the large firm ball is too intense on your forearm, you can use the large soft ball for this technique.

Friction

▶ *Using light, quick, random movements, rub the large firm ball between your hands in a scribbling motion. Be sure to include your fingers and wrists.*

LARGE SOFT BALL

Grip Reassess

Remember what your grip strength felt like when you began and repeat the Grip Assess with the large soft ball. Can you create a more powerful grip with less effort? Does your grip feel more equal from left to right?

Bonus Finger Techniques

Once you are familiar with the basic version of the Performance Hand Treatment, add these finger techniques. For athletes who need a strong grip, Knuckle Decompress with the small ball and Finger Rinsing will further improve grip strength and hand dexterity.

Knuckle Decompress

▶ *Place a small firm or soft ball between your index and middle fingers and bend your knuckles into your palm like you're making a fist. Squeeze the ball between your fingers in a slow pumping action 5 to 6 times.*

▶ *Place the ball between your middle and ring fingers, then between your ring and pinky fingers, and finally between your thumb and index finger, repeating the same compression and pumping action.*

▶ *Repeat on the other hand. This improves the sliding and gliding motion around the tendons.*

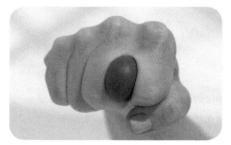

Finger Rinse

▶ *Place one hand down on a flat surface.*

▶ *Using the large soft ball, Rinse down your fingers from the base of your fingers to your fingertips.*

▶ *Repeat this over all of your fingers and your thumb.*

▶ *Repeat on the other hand.*

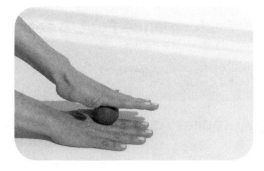

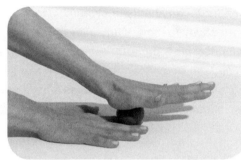

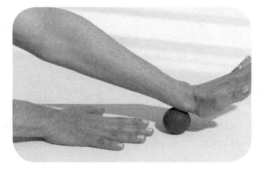

Mini Performance Hand Treatment

If you have limited time, you can do a Mini Performance Hand Treatment using just the large soft ball that will take fewer than 4 minutes. Use only these techniques in this order: Grip Assess, Glide, Direct and Indirect Shear, Finger Rinse, Friction, and Grip Reassess.

This quick treatment is great for game days, especially if you play a swing sport like golf, tennis, or baseball where rotational control and hand grip are essential.

▶ Performance Foot Treatment

You will need a large soft and a large firm ball.

Autopilot Assessments

When stuck stress interferes with your Autopilot's connection to your center of gravity, it can alter your overall balance and ground reaction force. This diminishes your ability to move with agility, good timing, and accuracy. You can identify whether this is compromising your overall stability with a standing assessment called the Body Scan Assess. Then test your Autopilot's efficiency with a Toe Lift Assess. Just like all of the MELT techniques, the setup is important.

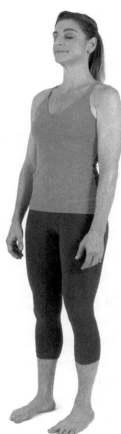

Body Scan Assess

Using Body Sense, you can identify if stuck stress is interfering with your Autopilot's connection to your center of gravity and its overall efficiency.

▶ *Stand upright. Line your feet up side by side, hip-width apart, toes facing forward. Place your hands at your side and close your eyes.*

▶ *Signs of stuck stress:*

– *Do you feel like you have more weight or surface area on one foot or you are sensing a region of either foot feeling more weighted into the ground?*

– *Scan up your legs. Notice whether you are clenching any muscles in your thighs or buttocks or locking out your knees. Can you release any muscles voluntarily yet still stay standing?*

▶ *Even though you put your feet side by side, do your legs and feet feel side by side? If it feels like one leg is staggered in front of the other or one leg feels rotated in or out compared with the other, those are also signs of Autopilot inefficiency.*

Toe Lift Assess

This assessment tests Autopilot efficiency by challenging your body to sustain connection to your center of gravity and the balance of your masses and spaces without the grip of your forefoot.

▶ *Stand upright, with feet hip-width apart. Close your eyes and lift all ten toes off the floor. Hold this position for 10 seconds to allow your Autopilot time to acquire connection to your center of gravity.*

▶ *Keep your eyes closed, take a breath in, and on the exhale, drop your toes back to the floor. Notice whether you feel your body drift or sway forward. That drift is a sign that your Autopilot is having trouble finding your center of gravity.*

▶ *Try the same assessment with your eyes open and notice how much less you drift when you can rely on your sense of sight to remain balanced compared to when you use only your Autopilot.*

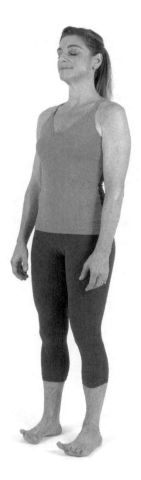

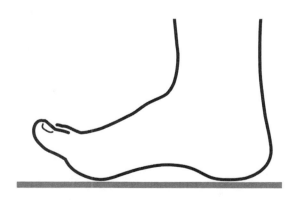

Position Point Pressing

▶ *Stand with your feet hip-width apart. With the large soft ball, step onto position point 1 at the center of your foot with a tolerable amount of pressure and take a focused breath.*

▶ *Shift your body weight from left to right, pumping the ball with compression slowly 5 to 10 times to find the right amount of tolerable pressure, and then compress and wait.*

▶ *To help your Autopilot acquire a better connection to your center of gravity, sustain the pressure on the ball and move your joints any way you want. Bring your arms over your head, wiggle your fingers, round your spine, bend your knees any random way, and then return to an upright position and take a focused breath.*

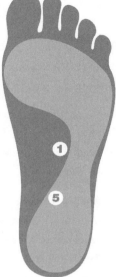

▶ *Step backward with the opposite foot and move the ball toward your heel by 1 inch to position point 5, directly in front of the heel pad. Gently rock your body weight forward by bending your knee slightly and apply tolerable compression to point 5. Pause for a moment, and then step back slightly to decompress and repeat one more time.*

Glide

▶ *With the ball at point 5, right in front of the heel, create a 50-50 split of your body weight.*

▶ *Your forefoot and toes should be on the floor, with your heel slightly lifted off the ground.*

▶ *Keeping your forefoot on the floor, slowly move your heel over the ball side to side in front of the heel for 15 seconds to find tolerable, consistent pressure.*

▶ *Continue Gliding the ball from side to side as you work your way to the back of the heel and then back to point 5.*

▶ *To get the most out of Gliding, keep the pressure constant as you move the ball from left to right under your foot.*

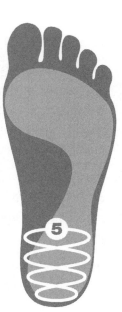

Direct Shear

▶ *With the large soft ball on point 5, sustain consistent pressure and wiggle your foot in very small movements left to right so the ball barely moves for approximately 15 to 20 seconds. Remember, Shearing requires friction and compression between the skin and the bones—so the ball isn't rubbing against your skin as much as you are pinning the flesh against the bones of your foot to induce the shear force. This is like working fluid into a sponge.*

▶ *Then stop moving, compress and hold the compression, and take two focused breaths as you allow the tissue to adapt. This is like squeezing a sponge out before you use it. Then decompress and take the ball out from under your foot.*

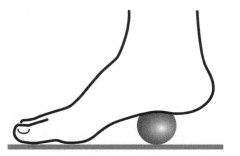

Foot Rinse

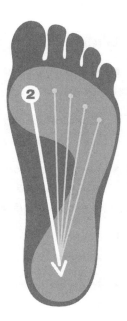

▶ *Practice Foot Rinsing with the large soft ball. Place the large soft ball under your big toe mound, point 2. Compress the knuckle to mobilize it, then keep the same pressure as you roll the ball toward your heel in a continuous one-directional motion with tolerable, consistent pressure.*

▶ *Shift your weight to your back foot and lift your front foot off the ball. Place the ball under the joint of your second toe, compress the joint, and repeat the rinsing pass from toe to heel.*

▶ *Repeat this motion from each toe to heel, shifting your weight on and off the ball between each pass.*

LARGE FIRM BALL

Next you'll repeat these techniques—Glide, Direct Shear, and Foot Rinse—on the same foot using the large firm ball. But first add an Indirect Shear at position point 1.

Indirect Shear

▶ *Stand with one foot in front of the other and place the large firm ball under point 1 of your front foot. Let your heel rest on the floor, toes relaxed over the ball. Soften your knee. Try to find equal weight on both feet. Keep your toes off the ground. Let your foot sink into the ball to create tolerable pressure.*

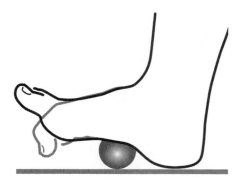

- Maintain consistent pressure as you curl your toes like a fist, then open and wiggle them.

- Repeat 3 times.

- Hold the compression and take two focused breaths as you allow the tissue to adapt.

Now repeat the Glide using the firm ball, but this time use it to investigate the tissue for stiffness. If you sense a lumpy texture or tenderness, this is what stuck stress feels like. Remember to be mindful with your pressure. Then repeat the Direct Shear and Rinse with the large firm ball.

Friction

- Using light, quick, random movements, balance on one foot and lightly rub your foot and toes over the ball in a scribbling motion. Allow your leg to be loose like a pendulum over the ball.

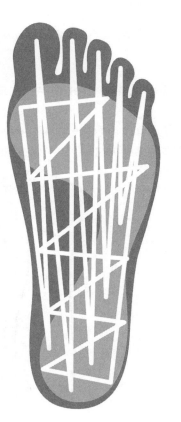

▶ Reassess

Body Scan Reassess

Place your feet side by side. You may notice that your feet feel different. I want you to learn what it feels like to sense fluid flow in your leg by using Body Sense. When joints are absent of fluid flow, you sense your joints more. On the leg you haven't MELTed yet, you may sense your hip, knee, or ankle joint. The leg you've done the treatment on, however, may feel more seamless and integrated.

▶ *Close your eyes. Do you notice any changes on the side of the body you treated?*

▶ *Scan your legs. Do you notice a difference in the joints of your legs and feet?*

Forward Bend Assess

If you're not sure what you feel using Body Sense, forward bend by rounding your spine, hinging at your hips, and reaching toward the floor.

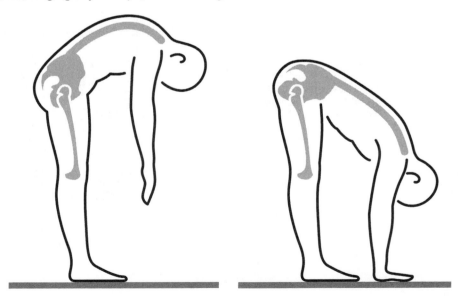

- *When fascia is hydrated, it gives muscles the opportunity to lengthen and stretch efficiently. Notice the leg you haven't MELTed yet. If your tissue is dehydrated, you'll notice that the pull is more segmented. You may feel tension in the tendons near your joints instead of a seamless pull.*

- *The leg you've hydrated may feel more seamless and the pull more integrated from foot to hip.*

Repeat the entire Foot Treatment using both balls on the other foot. At the end, alternate Friction on both feet, back and forth, two times before your final reassess. If you're ever short on time, you can just do Friction on both feet with the soft ball two times, as a quick treatment on its own to improve circulation.

Body Scan Reassess

Now that you've MELTed both feet, see whether you can identify improved efficiency in your Autopilot. Below are ideal changes that you may sense, which attest to improvement from your self-care.

- *Close your eyes and notice your footprints. Is your stance more equally weighted from left to right?*

- *Scan up your legs. If you started off feeling like you were contracting muscles unnecessarily and had to voluntarily relax, notice whether now you are naturally more efficient in your stance, legs feeling more side by side, with your eyes closed.*

Toe Lift Reassess

- *Keep standing with your eyes closed and lift all ten toes off the floor. You may notice that your body shifts back faster and you catch yourself more quickly than you did the first time. This is a good sign that new neurological information is being communicated throughout your body. Now your Autopilot needs time to organize this new information. This will occur as you start walking around or during your natural activities.*

▶ *Keep your eyes closed with your toes lifted, take a breath in, and on the exhale, drop your toes back to the floor. Do you drift less compared with your initial standing assessment?*

If you notice any of these changes, you are already sensing your ability to improve your whole-body efficiency just from treating your feet! You can do this treatment before or after any athletic training routine. It's also a great way to keep your feet in good condition and improve ankle stability and mobility. Both are essential for your overall longevity so use the Foot Treatment on its own or add it to any of the other sequences.

Mini Performance Foot Treatment

You can do a Mini Performance Foot Treatment by using just the large soft ball and working through the techniques in this order: Autopilot Assessments, Position Point Pressing, Glide, Direct Shear, Foot Rinse, and Friction. Take a moment to assess what happens when you treat just one foot to sense the changes you can make. Repeat it on the other side and then reassess.

▶ Upper Body Rehydrate Sequence

These are the foundational moves of the Upper Body Stability Sequence. Practice this sequence before adding the shoulder stability moves to get the most out of your self-care practice. There are five compression moves. The most basic is Upper Back Glide, Shear, and Rinse. If you are short on time, just do these techniques. On days when you have more time, add any or all of the other compression moves like Inner and Outer Shoulder Blade, Side Rib, Arm, and Chest to make greater and more lasting changes before you add the NeuroStrength moves in Chapter 7.

Rib Length Assess

Use Rib Length as a movement assessment before and after you do the compression moves instead of using the Rest Assess and Reassess. You can use some or all of the upper body compression moves (Upper Back, Inner Shoulder Blade, Rib and Outer Shoulder Blade, Arm and Chest Glide and Shear, and Upper Back Rinse) to build an upper body compression sequence. This will help reduce unnecessary tension and compression in your neck and low back space.

▶ *Bend your knees. Rest your shoulder blades on the roller.*

▶ *Interlace your fingers behind your head and let your neck relax. Your elbows are open and wide. Tuck your pelvis and remain in a tuck. Engage your core. As you create the following movement, your core, low back, and neck remain still and stable. Breathe in, and on the exhale, curl your ribs into flexion.*

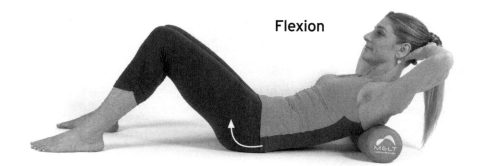

Flexion

▶ On the next exhale, engage your core and allow only your ribs to extend back over the roller and open your breastbone toward the ceiling. Your core, lower back, and neck maintain their position.

Extension

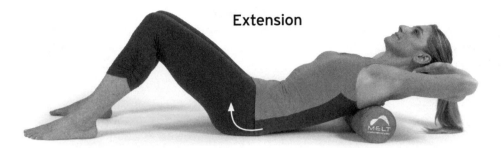

▶ Take two focused breaths into your ribs. Breathe in. On the exhale, curl your ribs forward and repeat the movement again.

▶ Next, try Rib Side Bending: From the extended position, breathe in, and on the exhale, slowly side bend your ribs to the right. Hold as you take a focused breath into the left side of your ribs. On your next exhale, return your torso to the center and then slowly side bend to the left. Hold as you take a focused breath into the right side of your ribs.

Side Bending

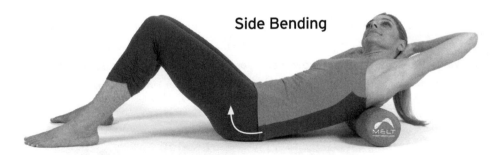

▶ Repeat 1 more time on each side. Notice whether you sense tension on either side or limitations in your range of movement. Remember what you feel. Return to this move after you do the compression moves below.

Upper Back Glide and Shear

▶ *Rest your upper back on the roller. Keep your hands behind your head for support, slightly curl your ribs forward, and point your elbows toward where the ceiling meets the wall ahead of you.*

▶ *Engage your core and lift your hips slightly off the floor, then move your hips toward your heels to bring the roller to the upper part of your back.*

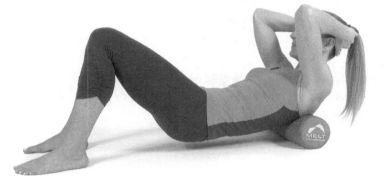

▶ *Begin Gliding by pushing into your feet to gently move the roller up and down just an inch or two, in a small area of your upper back 5 to 10 times to explore this region of your back for barriers or areas of sensitivity. Get smaller and smaller with your movements, and edge up against any area that feels a little sensitive, but don't land right on the most tender spot.*

▶ *Set your hips back down on the floor in a tucked position. Slightly curl your ribs forward and Shear the tissue by slowly side bending your upper body, tipping slightly left and right in small movements 3 to 4 times, as if you are twisting the flesh around one vertebra. Keep the pressure constant.*

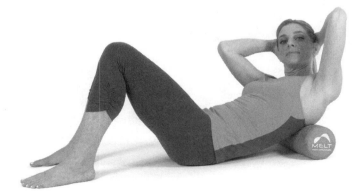

▶ *Return to the center, pause, and take a focused breath, letting your spine sink into the roller.*

▶ *Reset your feet and lift your hips slightly off the ground. Push into your feet to move the roller down your back 1–2 inches to another region near the bottom of your shoulder blades and repeat the Gliding motion to explore and prepare this region for the Shear.*

▶ *Find a spot where you can tolerate the pressure, get smaller and smaller with your movements, and then set your tucked pelvis back onto the floor. Curl your ribs slightly forward and repeat the Shear by tipping your torso slightly left and right a few times again. Pause and take a focused breath.*

You can do the following four moves on one side and then repeat on your other side. Or you can do each move on both sides, or pick a few instead of all four to try as a sequence.

Inner Shoulder Blade Glide and Shear

▶ *Rest your mid-back on the roller around the bottom of your shoulder blades with your hands behind your head, knees bent, and feet flat on the floor. Keeping your core engaged, tip your upper body slightly to the left and lift your hips slightly off the floor.*

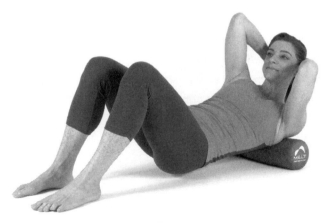

▶ *Begin the move with the roller on the bottom of your left shoulder blade, not on your spine. Keep your shoulders relaxed and back curled slightly forward, and*

begin Gliding. Using your feet, move the roller up and down the bottom edge of your shoulder blade. Notice whether it's tender. Move the roller up the inside edge of your shoulder blade 4 to 6 times. If you find a tender spot or a barrier, make your movement smaller and smaller and edge up against the area of stuck stress—don't land right on it.

▶ *Set your left buttock on the floor. To Shear, reach your arm out in front of you and move it up and down 5 to 10 times, keeping pressure on the inner shoulder blade to stimulate the tissue between your shoulder blade and shoulder joint.*

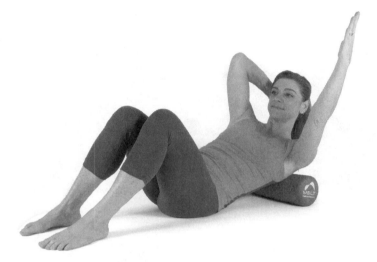

▶ Note: *If you have neck pain, keep your hand on your head and move your elbow toward your head and away from your head 5 to 10 times instead. If you have shoulder pain, place your hand on your shoulder and move your arm in front of your body in small circles 5 to 10 times with your elbow bent.*

▶ *Once you Shear, bring your hand back behind your head if you took it away; pause and wait. Take a focused breath.*

▶ *Return your body to the center. Repeat these steps on the other shoulder blade or, if you are using all of the techniques on one side at a time, continue to the Side Rib and Outer Shoulder Blade techniques.*

Side Rib Glide and Outer Shoulder Blade Glide and Shear

▶ *Lie on your left side with your mid-ribs, around the bra line, and your upper arm on the roller. Rest your head in your hand. Engage your core, hips on the ground.*

▶ *Glide on your side ribs by curling your torso into flexion and slightly back to extension 5 to 10 times. Investigate the tissue for tenderness or barriers. (You won't Shear your ribs.)*

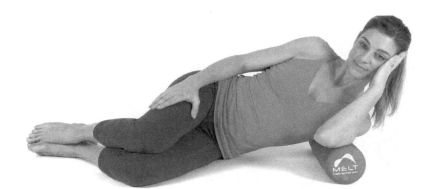

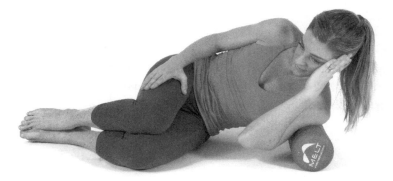

▶ *Glide your outer shoulder blade by slightly rotating your torso and left elbow toward the ceiling to bring the outer edge of your left shoulder blade on top of the roller. Gently side bend your torso to move the roller up and down the outside of the blade.*

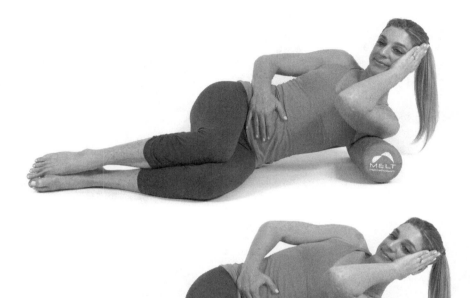

▶ *Keep the pressure constant. If you find a barrier, make your motion smaller and meet the barrier.*

▶ *Shear the shoulder blade by releasing your left arm and moving it like a rainbow up and over the top of the roller. The elbow stays bent.*

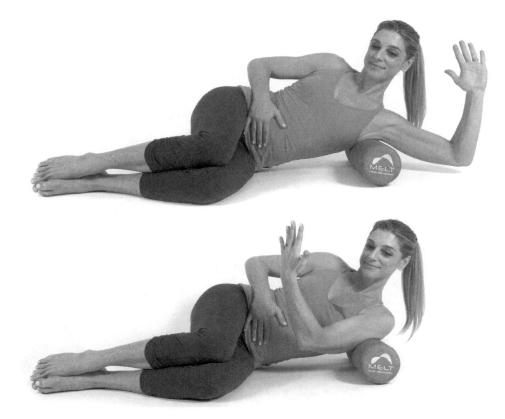

▶ *Return your hand to your head and take a focused breath, allowing the tissue to adapt.*

▶ *Repeat on the other side or continue to Arm Glide and Shear.*

Arm Glide and Shear

▶ *Lie on your side with your left upper arm on the roller at the bottom of your deltoid. If you grab your shoulder, your entire shoulder should be on the head side of the roller. The left elbow is bent, and the arm is relaxed on the floor.*

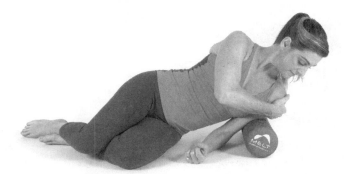

▶ *Use your top hand to support your head by placing your right forearm on the roller, palm faceup, and resting your head in your hand. Look toward the floor to reduce strain in the neck. Glide your arm by curling your upper body in and out slowly 5 to 10 times and explore this region for any areas of tenderness.*

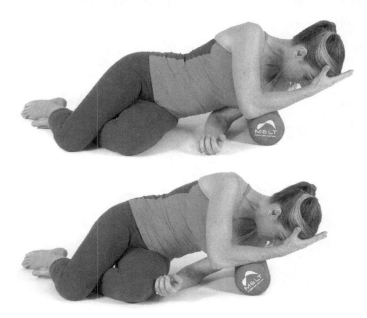

▶ *Find a spot where you can tolerate the pressure, pause on that spot, take a focused breath, and create an Indirect Shear by maintaining compression and rotating your left arm toward you and away from you 4 to 5 times as shown.*

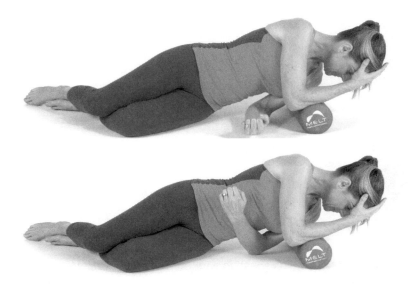

▶ Create a Direct Shear by resting your forearm on the floor and punching your arm forward and pulling back 4 to 5 times.

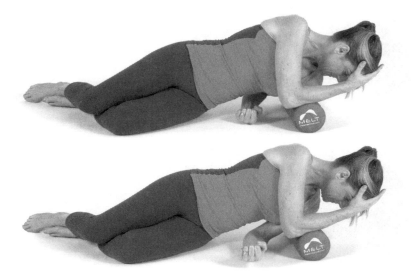

- *Take a focused breath and wait while you allow the tissue to adapt.*

- *Repeat on the other side or continue to Chest Glide and Shear.*

Chest Glide and Shear

- *Sit up and turn your torso toward the floor so your left arm is behind you, palm on the floor.*

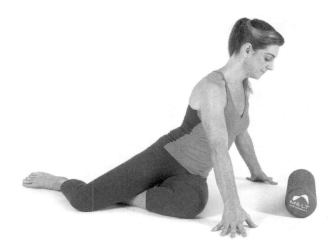

- *Rest the left upper arm bone and your chest, just below your collarbone, on the roller. Look toward the floor. If you feel any neck tension, support your head by resting your forehead in your right hand.*

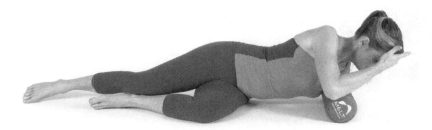

▶ *Use your hands and core to Glide the roller up and down the area below the collarbone by curling in toward your belly and extending the ribs slightly to sense your sternum and chest moving up and away from the floor. If your head is in your hand, you'll need to use your core more to curl your torso in and out to allow the roller to move properly.*

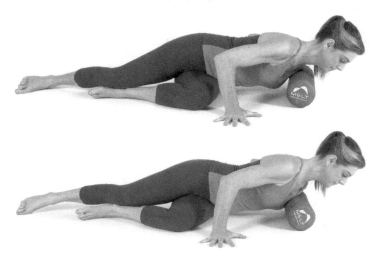

▶ *To Shear, create a cross-friction motion by moving the tissue between your skin and ribs left to right. Think of it like swiping back and forth on a smartphone or tablet. Pause, let your chest sink into the roller as you exhale, and allow the tissue to adapt.*

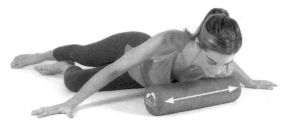

▶ *Repeat on the other side, or if you are using all of the techniques on one side at a time, return to the Inner Shoulder Blade Glide and Shear and repeat all of the techniques on the other side.*

After you have treated both sides, do the Upper Back Rinse to create a global fluid exchange throughout your entire body.

Upper Back Rinse

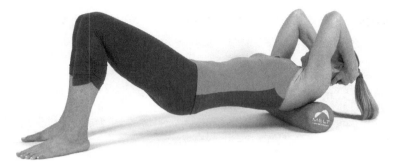

▶ *Find your core, set your feet slightly in front of your knees, and lift your hips 1 inch off the floor. Bring your knees over your ankles to move the roller to your upper back. Take a focused breath.*

▶ *On the exhale, engage your core, allow your hips to relax toward the floor slightly, and gently push into your feet to allow the roller to slowly travel down your rib region with consistent, light pressure. Curl your ribs forward slightly to sustain consistent pressure as your legs extend and your hips settle back to the floor.*

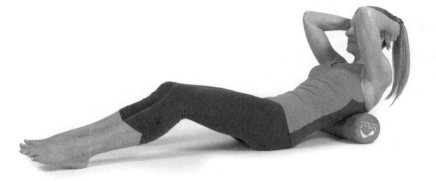

▶ *Reset your feet slightly in front of your knees and then find your core, lift your hips off the floor, and bring your knees over your feet again so the roller moves to your upper back. Pause and take a focused breath.*

▶ *Repeat the Rinse 3 to 4 times to improve fluid flow throughout your body.*

Rib Length Reassess

Reassess your ability to move your ribs to see if you've improved your range of motion.

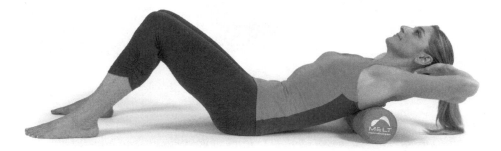

▶ *Bend your knees. Rest your shoulder blades on the roller. Interlace your fingers behind your head and relax your neck. Your elbows are open and wide. Tuck your pelvis and remain in a tuck. Engage your core. As you create the following movement, your core, low back, and neck remain still and stable.*

▶ *Breathe in, and on the exhale, curl your ribs into flexion. On the next exhale, engage your core, allow only your ribs to extend over the roller, and open your breastbone toward the ceiling. Your core, lower back, and neck maintain their positions.*

▶ *Take two focused breaths into your ribs. Breathe in. On the exhale, curl your ribs forward into flexion and again slowly extend to the Rib Length position.*

▶ *This time, from the extended position, breathe in, and on the exhale, slowly side bend your ribs to the right. Hold as you take a focused breath into the left side of your ribs.*

▶ *On your next exhale, return your torso to the center and then slowly side bend to the left. Hold as you take a focused breath into the right side of your ribs.*

▶ *Repeat 1 more time on each side.*

▶ *Notice whether you have increased range of motion or whether both sides of your rib region can move more freely.*

▶ Lower Body Rehydrate and Low Back Release Sequence

Begin this sequence with a basic Rest Assess and end with a Rest Reassess so that you can value the direct and indirect changes this sequence can make in the positions of your masses and spaces. Don't forget to also check your ability to turn your head left and right. You might find that the Lower Body Rehydrate Sequence indirectly improves your neck range of motion as well as your Autopilot's connection to your center of gravity.

These are the foundational moves of the NeuroCore Stability Sequence. Practice this sequence on its own before trying the NeuroCore moves and ultimately the full stability sequence.

Rest Assess

▶ *Notice your masses and spaces. What common imbalances do you notice using Body Sense before you begin the sequence?*

▶ *Make a note of what you feel in your alignment, your ability to turn your head, and your Autopilot's ability to find your center of gravity. Remember what you feel.*

Differentiation: Tuck and Tilt Your Pelvis

For length moves, your pelvis will have to either be in a tuck or a tilt. Let's practice these two moves now so you can focus on sustaining these positions to get the most out of the lower body length moves.

Note: It's essential that you differentiate your pelvis from your legs and ribs, so tune in to what's staying stable as you try to move your pelvis from the tuck to the tilted position. Remember, the movement is subtle and controlled. Your range of movement can be small. By controlling this movement while keeping your other masses still, you will reconnect your Autopilot to your center of gravity and enhance its control and connection.

Modified Tuck and Tilt Challenge

▶ *Engage your core, lift your hips, and place the center of your pelvis on top of the roller. The top of your hip bones should be on the torso side of the roller, not on top of the roller. Your low back should not be on the roller.*

▶ *Place your feet on the floor, hip width apart. First, tuck your pelvis. Your pubic bone will curl toward your navel and you'll sense your low back lengthen. Keep your feet light on the floor rather than pressing into your feet to acquire the tuck.*

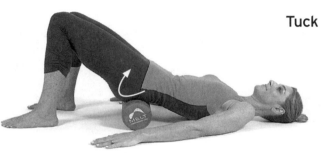

Tuck

▶ *Remain in the tuck and take a focused breath. Notice the weight of your mid ribs on the floor. Without moving your ribs from this position, try to untuck your pelvis back to the top of the roller. Your pubic bone will move away from your navel, and your low back curve will lift back to its neutral arch. This position is the tilt.*

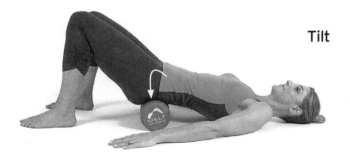

Tilt

▶ *Move your pelvis from the tucked to the tilted position 5 to 10 times without pushing your feet into the floor or moving your ribs. This is called differentiated motion. Focus on where you want to stay still rather than what's moving to improve your Autopilot's connection to your center of gravity.*

SI Joint Shear

▶ *Engage your core, lift your hips, and place the center of your pelvis on top of the roller. The center of your pelvis is on the roller. Your low back should not be on the roller. Find your core as you bring your thighs toward your chest, stopping just past the roller, heels to the buttocks as shown.*

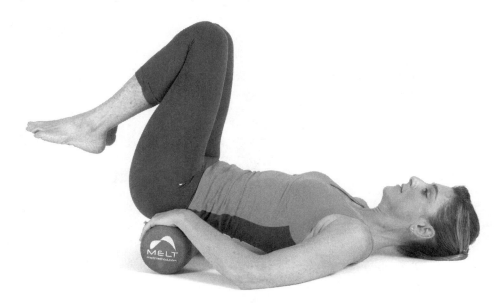

▶ *Slowly tip your legs left and right and slide your hands under your outer hips to prevent tipping too far so you stay on your sacrum and SI joints rather than tipping onto your outer hip. Try to keep your knees together to reduce strain to your low back. Pause on the left SI Joint.*

▶ *There are three ways to Shear the SI joint. (1) The easiest is to slowly march your knees forward and back 3 to 4 times staying on the angle. (2) You can also make small circles in either direction with the leg you're leaning toward while keeping the other leg still. The movement comes from your hip joint while your pelvis and ribs stay stable. (3) Or you can keep your knees together and circle both legs at the same time while you sustain a slight angle with your legs to one side. Then, keep your legs tipped to the left side, pause for a moment, maintain the pressure, and take two focused breaths to give the tissue time to adapt.*

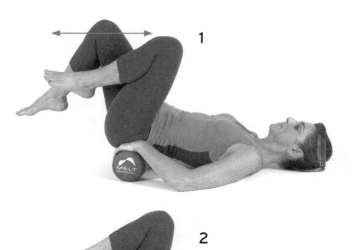

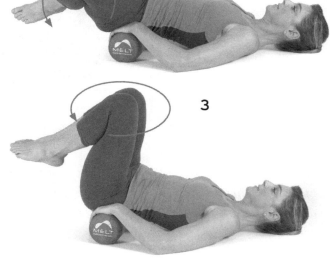

▶ *Return your knees to the center and repeat on the right side.*

▶ *You can use one, two, or all three movements to improve stability and hydration to your pelvis.*

Bent Knee Press

▶ *With the roller still under your pelvis, place your left foot on the floor and bring your right leg toward your chest as shown. Tuck your pelvis and allow your ribs to relax and sink into the floor. Engage your core.*

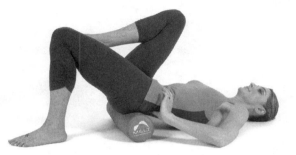

▶ *Interlace your fingers over your right shin or around the back of your thigh. Keep your left foot firmly on the floor and keep your left knee in line with your hip. Don't let it swing out to the left side of your body. Make sure your hips remain square and level on top of the roller from left to right.*

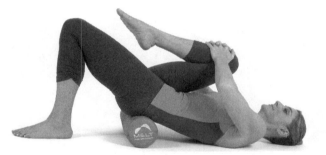

▶ *Inhale, and on the exhale, accentuate the tuck of your pelvis and energize your left knee over your toes as you tuck your pelvis toward your nose to sense the tensional length along the front of your left thigh.*

▶ *Inhale again, and then exhale and tuck the pelvis as you draw your right knee toward your torso again to accentuate the tensional pull along the front of your left thigh. Think about your left knee reaching over your left foot in the opposite direction.*

▶ *Take a focused breath. Set your right foot on the floor, and repeat this lengthening technique on the right thigh.*

Hip to Heel Press

▶ *Keep your right foot light on the floor, pelvis in an active tilt on top of the roller. Extend your left leg as shown.*

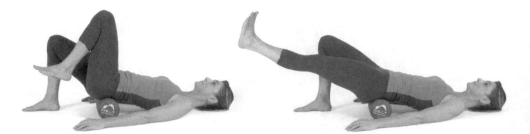

▶ *Focus on keeping your knee fully extended, pelvis remains in an active tilt, ribs heavy, as you begin to slowly flex your hip joint and move your leg toward perpendicular.*

▶ *Stop before your leg passes perpendicular to the roller or starts to bend at the knee.*

▶ *Once you sense tension on the back of your leg, accentuate the pelvic tilt and flex your foot again.*

▶ *Take two focused breaths, enhancing the tensional length from hip to heel on each exhale, and then release your left foot to the floor, with the knee bent.*

▶ *Repeat on the right leg.*

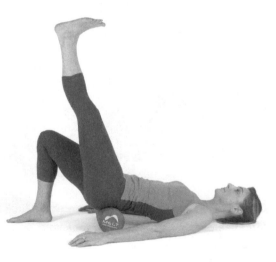

Figure 4

▶ *Place your left foot on the floor with your left knee bent. Flex your right ankle and cross it over the left thigh by the left knee. Breathe in. On the exhale, find your core as you bring your legs into your chest. Notice the stretch you create on the back of your right hip. Although that's a great sensation, now we want to restore hydration around your hip joint.*

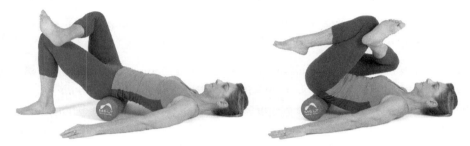

▶ *Place your left hand either on your right foot or behind the left thigh. Place your right hand on the front of your right thigh. Slowly push your legs away from you until your left leg is perpendicular to the roller. Your left thigh should be as close to perpendicular to the roller as possible. Your right knee remains bent,*

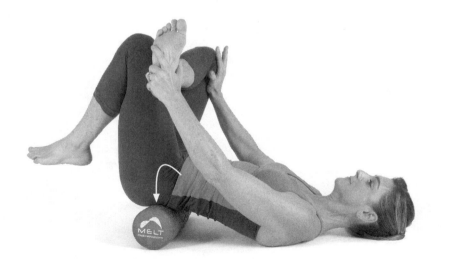

and your right ankle remains flexed. Keep the pelvis level and avoid lateral tilting.

▶ *At the same time, with equal intensity in opposing directions, use your right hand to press your right thigh up (imagining it moving away from the hip socket) and forward gently. In opposition, to acquire the two-directional length, gently press your left thigh into your right ankle (as if you want to bring your left knee toward your chest) to accentuate the external rotation of the right hip joint. This encourages tensional length around the right hip joint. Your pelvis should remain still throughout this move. Don't let your pelvis laterally tip or rotate while creating this tensional length.*

▶ *Once this "push-press" position is achieved, take a focused breath and actively tilt the pelvis on the top of the roller without lifting your ribs from the floor. Inhale and decrease the three compression points slightly. On the exhale, tilt your pelvis on top of the roller without arching your back as you press your left knee toward your right ankle and push your right knee away from your hip joint. Take a focused breath.*

▶ *Set your left foot back on the floor, release your right leg, and repeat on the other side.*

Pelvic Tuck and Tilt Challenge

▶ *Bring both knees toward your chest. Place your palms on the front of your thighs, close to your knees. Gently push your knees away from your chest until your arms are straight. Keep your thighs angled slightly toward your torso to avoid any unnecessary tension on your low back, and try to keep your shoulders relaxed and unshrugged.*

▶ *Take a focused breath and actively sink your ribs toward the floor below your shoulder blades and gently press your thighs into your hands as if you were trying to bring your knees to your chest, but don't bend your elbows or shrug your shoulders. You shouldn't move at all; rather, you should sense a deep abdominal contraction. These are the powerful muscles that stabilize the lumbar spine.*

▶ *Once you are in this position, take a breath in, and on the exhale, try to tuck your pelvis, sensing your pubic bone curling toward your navel without moving your thighs forward; then, while sustaining the pressure of your thighs toward your hands, slowly tilt your pelvis to return the back side of your pelvis and sacrum to the top of the roller. Notice whether your ribs come with you. If they do, make the movement smaller to differentiate your pelvis from your legs and torso.*

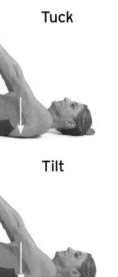

Tuck

Tilt

▶ *Repeat the tuck and tilt movements 4 to 5 times, moving slowly; exhale each time you tuck and tilt the pelvis.*

   – *If this move is too challenging, place your feet on the floor and practice the Modified Tuck and Tilt Challenge (page 160) to improve pelvic control.*

Low Back Decompress

▶ *Sustain three points of compression: your pelvis in the tilted position on top of the roller, your thighs gently pressing into your hands, and your ribs relaxed and heavy on the floor.*

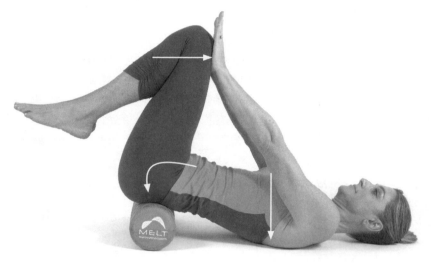

▶ *Inhale, and on an exhale, accentuate the three points of compression and find your core by either forcing your exhale with a* shhh, ssss, *or* haaa *sound or just by taking a focused exhale.*

▶ *Try this 3 times and then slowly bring both knees into your chest, roll the roller out from under your pelvis, and reassess your masses and spaces by lying on the floor with your arms and legs extended.*

Rest Reassess

▶ *Lie on the floor with your arms and legs straight and relaxed, palms faceup. Breathe and allow your body to relax into the floor. Close your eyes and take a moment to reassess.*

▶ *Using your Body Sense, notice your masses and spaces. Remember the common imbalances you identified before you tried this sequence. Are your lower body masses feeling more weighted? Is your pelvis more weighted on your butt cheeks rather than on your tailbone? Have the backs of your thighs settled to the floor? Is your low back curve more relaxed and, ideally, feeling more lifted closer to your pelvis? Do your ribs feel more weighted to the floor?*

▶ *Turn your head from left to right. Do you have more range of motion? Is there less pain or stiffness as you turn your head?*

▶ *Assess your Autopilot. Do the left and right sides of your body feel more evenly weighted? Does it feel like there's less of a distinction between the left and right halves of your body?*

▶ *Finally, take a full breath and notice what areas of your torso expand when your lungs fill with air. Do you sense greater movement? Is it easier to take a deep breath?*

▶ *Remember, noticing changes not only allows you to identify whether your self-care has had an effect but allows your Autopilot to reset and acquire better neurological connection to your center of gravity.*

❱ Seated Compression Sequence

Begin this sequence with a Rest Assess and end with a Rest Reassess so that you can value the direct and indirect changes this sequence can make. Don't forget to also check your ability to turn your head left and right. You might find that the Seated Compression Sequence indirectly improves your neck range of motion as well as your Autopilot's connection to your center of gravity.

These are the foundational moves of the Lower Body Stability Sequence. Practice this sequence on its own before trying the Lower Body Stability moves and ultimately the full Lower Body Stability Sequence.

Deep Hip Glide and Shear

❱ *Sit on the roller, knees bent. Place your hands on the floor in front of the roller. Glide back and forth over your sits bones.*

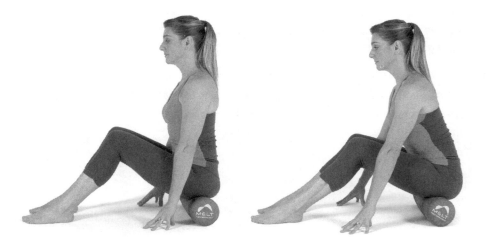

▶ *Place your left hand on the floor behind the roller to support some of your body weight and your right hand on your knees as you Glide on and around your left sits bone. Notice whether there is tenderness on one sits bone or whether the bone flips over the roller as you Glide over and around it.*

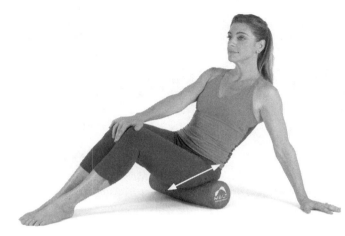

▶ *Once you feel balanced and can coordinate the motion of your body over the roller, keep your core engaged and drop your left knee toward the floor. Relax the leg in this position and continue to Glide the deep hip 6 to 10 times using your right leg and your core to navigate your body weight over the roller. Keep your left hand light on the floor to avoid shoulder tension. Gently Glide up and down, making your moves smaller and smaller when you sense a barrier. You can also create small circular motions around the side of your hip. Meet the barrier and take a focused breath.*

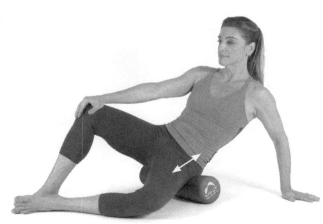

▶ *Create an Indirect Shear by moving your knee up and down, creating rotation at the hip joint 3 to 4 times.*

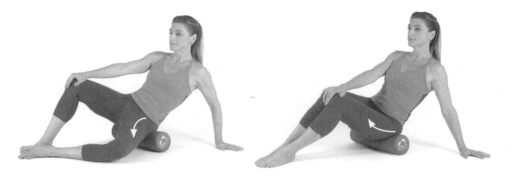

▶ *Create a Direct Shear by straightening out the left knee and allowing your body to move over the roller 3 to 4 times. (Do not create a cross-friction motion in this region of the hip, which could irritate the sciatic nerve.)*

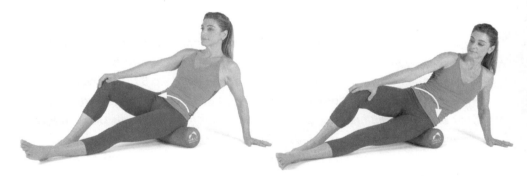

▶ *Take a focused breath and wait while you allow the tissue to adapt.*

▶ *Slowly return to the top of the roller, lean to the other side, and repeat, beginning with your knees angled upward.*

Tail Triangle and SI Joint Glide

▶ *Position the roller at the center of your sacrum, at the back of your pelvis. Place your arms wide behind you with your fingers pointed outward, elbows bent, core engaged, buttocks relaxed, and knees bent. Keep your shoulders relaxed.*

▶ *Actively tuck your pelvis and think of your hands and feet remaining light on the floor to activate your core. Ribs should be slightly flexed. Breathe in.*

▶ *On the exhale, Glide up and down the sacrum 6 to 10 times.*

▶ *Next, bring your feet together, tip your knees slightly to the left, and continue Gliding. You are now on your left SI joint. Keep your arms wide behind you with your fingers pointed outward, elbows bent, core engaged, and buttocks relaxed. Keep your shoulders relaxed. Keep the pelvis in a slight tuck with your core engaged.*

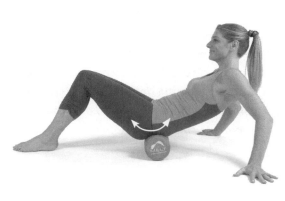

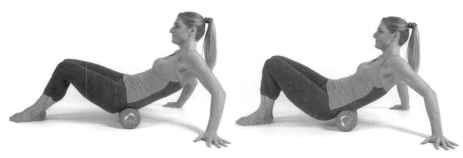

▶ *Glide over the left SI joint 6 to 10 times using your core and legs (rather than your arms) to control the speed and movement of the roller.*

▶ *Repeat the Glide on the right SI joint by tipping your knees a little to the right. Take note of which side is more tender. You can repeat the Glide on the tender side an extra time before trying the next move.*

Side Hip Glide and Shear

▶ *Place your left forearm on the floor behind the roller, knees bent, with the roller on the side of your pelvis, below the top of your hip and above the top of the thigh bone. Keep your shoulder relaxed and your core engaged.*

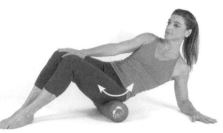

▶ *You can place your right hand on your top knee. Breathe in. Exhale and Glide over the side of your hip by gently rolling up and down using your right leg and your core. With the right knee pointed toward the ceiling, lower the left knee to the floor and continue to Glide. When you find a barrier, make your Glide movements smaller and smaller and meet the barrier.*

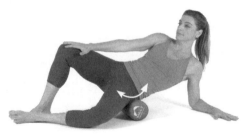

▶ *Create an Indirect Shear by rotating at the hip joint, moving your thigh toward the floor and back together 3 to 4 times.*

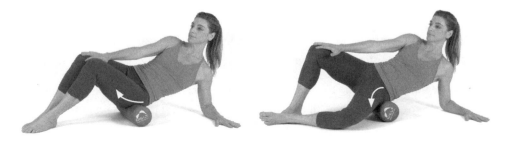

◗ *Create a Direct Shear by straightening out your left leg and rolling left to right while sustaining compression 3 to 4 times.*

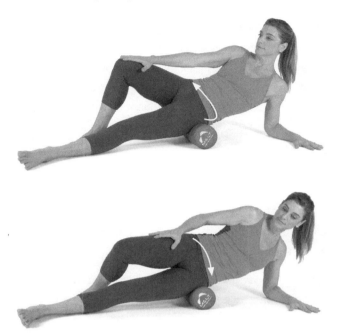

◗ *If it feels like you're going over a speed bump, try cross-friction—shifting your pelvis forward and back 3 to 4 times over the roller to twist the flesh around your pelvis.*

◗ *Take a focused breath and wait while you allow the tissue to adapt.*

◗ *Find your core as you lift your torso up and turn over to repeat on the other side.*

▌ Neck Release Sequence

You can do this sequence all on its own or add it to any of the stability sequences to improve the freedom of your neck and improve performance. Don't forget to Rest Assess and Rest Reassess your masses and spaces as well as your current ability to turn your head. You may also find that adding this sequence alleviates many of the other common imbalances and gives the stability sequences a boost in results. The base of your skull is full of sensory receptors, so this sequence can quickly improve your Autopilot's efficiency and control.

Neck Turn Assess

▌ *Lie on your back with your arms and legs extended. Scan your masses and spaces for stuck stress and any common imbalances.*

▌ *Turn your head left and right, and notice whether you have limited range or pain or whether your shoulders move as you turn your head.*

▌ *Take a moment to notice your left- and right-side balance. Remember, if your Autopilot has a good connection to your center of gravity, you'll feel balanced from left to right. If you feel offset to one side, make a note of this before you begin the sequence.*

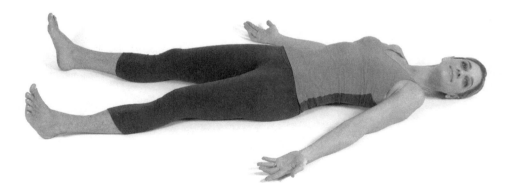

Base of Skull Shear

▶ *Lie on your back with your knees bent, and place the roller at the base of your skull by tipping your chin up slightly as you rest your head on the roller. To ensure that you have the roller in the right place, touch your hairline at the nape of your neck. It should be on the curved part of the roller, not on top of the roller.*

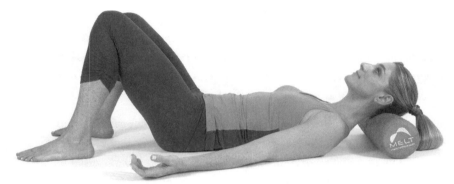

▶ *Slowly turn your head left and right. If the roller is in the right position, it will remain still. If it slides into your neck space, you started with the roller too close to your neck space; if it slips out from under your head, you're dropping your chin as you turn your head.*

▶ *Once you have the roller in the proper position, drop your left leg out to the side and allow your head to angle slightly to the left.*

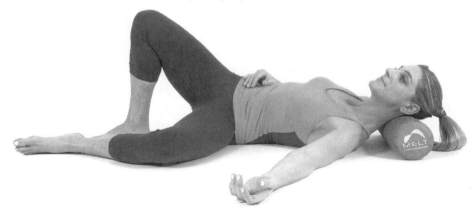

▶ *Relax your shoulders and Shear by making small circles 4 to 6 times with your head and breathe into the area you are compressing. Now make a few circles 4 to 6 times in the opposite direction. To create cross-friction, slowly turn your head a little left and right. Imagine keeping your skin pinned to the roller and allowing your skull to rub against the inside of your flesh. Think of crimping or wrinkling the tissue behind your ear as your head turns toward the roller and pulling it taut as you turn your nose slightly away from the roller.*

▶ *Now pause, wait, and take a focused breath.*

▶ *Slowly return your body to the center, reach out your right arm, and allow your right leg to relax outward on the floor. Shear the right side of the base of your skull with small circles in both directions or with small head turning. Keep your movements small and controlled. Pause, wait, and take a focused breath.*

▶ *After you've done both sides, lie on your back with your knees bent, and return the center of the base of your skull to the roller. Lift your chin slightly. While maintaining consistent pressure, create small figure eight motions on the center of the base of your skull. I imagine a movement of my skull like a backstroke, rolling the base of my skull up and over the top of the roller 5 to 6 times. Keep the pressure constant and your chin slightly lifted.*

▶ *Stop, wait, and take a focused breath to give the tissue time to adapt.*

Neck Decompress

▶ *Place your hands on the roller, tip your nose up as if you were trying to look straight up at the ceiling, and move the roller up about 1 inch toward the center of the back of your head.*

▶ *Once you have the roller in place, take your hands away and try to sustain this position with gentle pressure on the top of the roller at the center of the back of your head.*

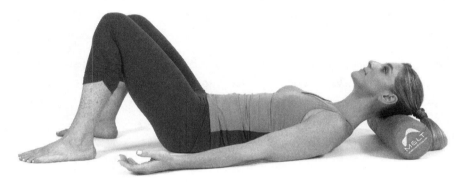

▶ *Inhale, and on the exhale, slowly nod your chin slightly toward your chest, but don't lose your neck space.*

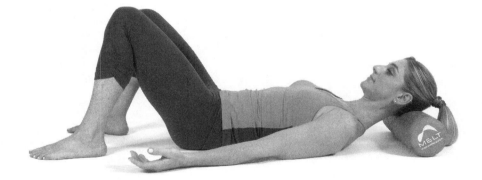

▶ *Pause in this position, keep the pressure the same, inhale as you hold this position, and on the exhale, tip your nose and chin back up toward the ceiling as if you were smelling something good in the air or kissing someone slightly taller than you. Pause in this position, inhale, and as you exhale, nod your nose down again.*

▶ *Repeat this head nod 4 times, pausing on the inhale, moving on the exhale. Then, remove the roller from the back of your head, and gently bring your head to the floor to reassess.*

Neck Turn Reassess

▶ *Lie on your back with your arms and legs extended. You may notice that your neck space feels more lifted and open. Sensing heat in the neck is also a common sensation and indicates restored blood flow and hydration. Turn your head left and right and notice whether you have increased range of motion or less pain.*

▶ *Improving the stability of your neck can make global changes, so notice your masses and spaces. Even though you didn't do anything to your low back, does releasing your neck also change the tension in your low back or improve your Autopilot's connection to your center of gravity? Do you feel more balanced from left to right?*

After you've tried the Rehydrate and Release sequences, you will probably be aware of how quickly you can make changes in your body and bring it back to balance.

Learning to use Body Sense is something new. For some people it comes easily, whereas others will question what they feel again and again. Some clients say they don't feel anything. What they don't realize, until I point it out, is that "feeling nothing" is to some extent impossible. You aren't feeling "nothing"—you simply aren't sure what change feels like at that moment. Self-care truly is the best care when it comes to resilience, but it takes practice and repetition, just like any sports training. You must condition your mind and invite yourself to sense what's going on inside the body, such as unnecessary tension and being able to consciously relax. Sensing subtle changes in your body can in fact make massive changes in your function and how you then perceive, act, and learn.

Change, no matter how small, is vital to your longevity. Your world feels small and frustrating when you try to change and don't think you can. I get that. But you *do* have it in you to harness the changeability self-care can create. Practice not perfection is my mantra. You are simply looking to identify your body's baseline. Assess, then reassess. Make a note which sequences have notable effects. Don't toss out sequences that you don't think make much change, because you'll soon learn that putting NeuroStrength moves into these sequences is the magic ingredient that will restore stability and allow you to sense bigger changes.

Remember, the question shouldn't be how long it will take for you to feel better—it should be, *How little can I do to sense a change in the right direction?* Small steps get you to a new place far faster than taking one haphazard leap.

6

Reintegrate and Repattern
The Two Rs of NeuroStrength

The heart of the MELT Method is treating connective tissue dehydration, or stuck stress, which accumulates and causes four common imbalances that if left unaddressed cause unnecessary tension or compression in the neck or low back, leading to chronic pain.

With the Four Rs of MELT—Reconnect, Rebalance, Rehydrate, and Release—you have the tools to improve the function and stability of your fascia. By rehydrating your connective tissue, you improve the environment of the sensorimotor pathways, and your joints and muscles have the space and connection they need to create better movement. When fascia is healthy, it anticipates how you want to move, and pre-stresses muscles and joints so you move efficiently. Aside from fascia there are muscles that contract specifically to *stabilize* a joint and then other muscles *move* the joint.

This is what the Two Rs of NeuroStrength—Reintegrate and Repattern—are here to help you restore. I'm going to teach you how to restore the neurological pathways and natural timing of the motor response needed for stability during movement. These Two Rs will give you the stable, efficient movement necessary for an active, pain-free lifestyle.

As you learned in Chapter 1, primal patterns—our basic motor programs—are developed in the womb and then hardwired up until the age of two. These are the basic patterns we continue to use to stabilize and move us during our lives. But as we develop habitual postures and movements, we begin to adopt compensatory patterns—even when we think we're exercising and moving with proper form. Injury, pregnancy, and aging all contribute to compensatory stability and motion as well. The natural, integrated stabilizing pathways become altered, and how we stabilize and move our body begins to change.

A perfect example of this happened in the gym a few years ago when a body builder came to me for advice. He told me that his shoulder hurt every time he did a bench press. I showed him how to do a quick MELT Hand Treatment and a shoulder stabilization technique, and then told him to do his press. He picked up the 325 barbell, let out a "Whoa!," quickly put it back, and sat up as I asked him whether he was okay. "I thought you lightened the weight!" he said.

"I didn't," I said with a smile. "Go on, do your one rep max bench press."

Instead of doing one, he easily did three, and then looked at me in amazement.

"What did you *do*?" he asked. "It's *magic*!"

"It's not magic," I told him. "We're just triggering a change in your nervous system. Before, as soon as you bent your elbow, your shoulder joint looked compromised and unstable, and your muscles were firing in a faulty pattern. We rehydrated your connective tissue, then diverted your brain's attention with Reintegration techniques, and got the faulty pattern out before you did the movement again. The difference was that your shoulder girdle was more stable, and your brain used a new neural pathway to move your arms."

"But the *movement's* the same," he said, looking perplexed.

"Yes and no. It might look the same, but the stability and control to execute the movement improved when you had to move the weight down to your chest, so it was easier for you to press it back up," I answered, knowing he wouldn't quite get it.

His eyes lit up. "So am I stronger now?" he asked.

"Not really stronger; you're just more stable so you're not compensating so much now. Your muscle timing improved, so I guess you feel it's easier to press the weight because your shoulder joint is in a better place," I explained to him.

I knew he got it because then he said, "That's kind of amazing it worked so fast. Should I be doing this stuff before I weight train?"

"Yes! If you spend just ten minutes stabilizing your shoulder before you train, you'll improve your performance and decrease your risk of damaging your shoulder joint."

He had felt the nearly instantaneous power of MELT Performance.

This is what Reintegration and Repatterning are all about: restoring proper neural pathways for the deep stabilizing mechanisms in your body to activate properly. Although stability is normally achieved without our conscious control, these techniques teach you how to reopen the pathways and reactivate the mechanisms of stability. It's all about setting up the position to give your brain a chance to reboot a proper stabilizing pathway before you create any movement.

In this chapter, I explain the how and why of Reintegration and Repatterning, as these techniques *always* work in tandem—they're the two integral steps of MELT Performance. Repatterning without reintegrating the proper neurological pathways first only creates more compensation. You'll learn to identify and sense in your body when you are in the correct position for Reintegration. The secret sauce is giving your stability mechanisms this reboot before you repattern the movement.

Reintegration and Repatterning help your body become more stable when you move during every activity you do. The muscles of your arms and legs will be recruited more efficiently; you'll be able to maintain pelvic and shoulder girdle balance, integrity, and stability during movement; you will improve dynamic agility in all directions; and your joints will experience less compression, which means more energy, less pain, and improved performance.

You'll soon find out what makes these Two Rs work so well once you start doing the moves in the following chapter. Almost anyone can do the basic moves, at any age or fitness level, to achieve better stability and motor control.

▶ About Stabilizing Mechanisms

Before I go into detail about Reintegration and Repatterning, it's important to learn about the basics of your pelvic and shoulder stability mechanisms, because this is key to understanding why the Two Rs work so well to improve your performance.

I've found that the word *mechanism* tends to trip people up when learning about stability. But it's really just the difference between involuntary, slow-twitch muscle fibers and voluntary, fast-twitch muscle fibers that separates stabilizing potential and movement potential. Stability mechanisms provide involuntary, neurological, sensorimotor control potential. What's compelling is how the brain sends information to the muscles, whether we move or not. When we move, we must ideally first be stable so we don't compromise our joints. That's the point of stability. We don't think about it; we just do what we do and move when we want to go somewhere.

Pelvic and shoulder stability mechanisms "anticipate" our movements. The involuntary, deep, slow-twitch muscles closest to the joints create stability. We don't have

Pelvis and Shoulders: The Two Primary Girdles

Recent research has focused on how sensorimotor control is acquired by pelvic stability. Focusing on the pelvis (the body's center of gravity in upright posture) rather than the spine will ideally lead to better treatments for back pain. This new research addresses three primary elements: structure (form or anatomy), function (sensorimotor control), and the mind (emotions and awareness when discussing human performance and stability). One of the reasons it's hard to do this kind of research on how much movement is optimal is because everyone's pelvis is anatomically unique; and age, pregnancy, and one's history often have distinct effects on the pelvis as well.

What's important for you to know now is that the two primary girdles that give your body stability are the pelvic girdle and the shoulder girdle. And they aren't called girdles for nothing—just as women used to lace themselves into girdles for abdominal support, these girdles give your body the support it needs so your arms and legs can move freely.

The pelvic and shoulder girdles support your limbs as you move. You take this for granted: Whether how you move is as simple as lifting your arm to open a door or as complicated as dancing for a ballet company, learning how to reintegrate stability and repattern primary motor patterns will allow your spine, arms, and legs to move more efficiently.

The most unique part of MELT Performance is understanding the Indirect Before Direct approach to improving stability in a girdle. For example, the starting place to improve your shoulder stability and agility—so that you'll be able to swing a tennis racket as you want to and without pain, for example—is to establish better neurological timing and motor control in your *hips*. A tennis swing doesn't come from the arms; it comes from the feet up. So if your pelvis isn't stable, you can't rotate your torso to gain the velocity and accuracy needed to swing the racket. Your shoulder gets strained but the issues are perhaps caused by pelvic instability and the compensation that starts before you even move your arms.

As you'll see in Part Three, the MELT Performance Lower Body Stability Sequence can improve the accuracy and power of your tennis swing. Once your hips and ground reaction force are more efficient, you can add the Upper Body Stability Sequence to improve precision and power.

much conscious control over this process during motion, but we can access the control of these muscles if we know how.

Here's an example of stabilizing and moving the shoulder. A key rotator cuff muscle called the supraspinatus ideally activates to draw the head of the humerus, or arm bone, into the shoulder socket a moment before the muscle mover, your lateral deltoid, contracts along with other muscles to lift your arm out to the side. In this instance, the supraspinatus would be the stabilizer of the shoulder joint, and the deltoid would be considered the agonist or muscle that moves the limb upward and away from the side of the body. If the supraspinatus doesn't activate, you still move your arm, but you compensate to do it and this compensation can go unnoticed. When I evaluate my clients with this simple movement, often I see them shrug or elevate their shoulder, slightly tip their head, side bend subtly at the waistline, and voilà, they lift their arm. They don't realize that the movement is faulty because they moved their arm when I asked them to. When you do repetitive movements, compensation can arise whether you know it or not—especially when you train for a specific sport.

By improving the stability mechanisms, Reintegration and Repatterning will improve the timing of the stabilizers so your function will be improved and your movements will be more precise.

What Can Inhibit These Stabilizers?

There are several different reasons why stabilizers can become inhibited:

- *Connective tissue dehydration*, causing imbalance and weakness. This tends to be a primary cause of imbalance in the first place, leading to poor motor patterns. When fascia loses its elastic properties and supportive qualities, sensorimotor function can become delayed, thus movement efficiency declines on every level.

- *Overuse, misuse, and disuse of muscles, and, of course, aging,* cause muscular imbalance, which can cause certain dominant muscles to shorten while others become lengthened. If a muscle is not able to contract or release when we try to move, pain, joint compression, and compensation occur. It doesn't matter if a muscle is locked long or short; in both states it can become inhibited or weak in motor response. Short, tight muscles aren't necessarily "strong." In either state they lose their adaptability and ability to respond. Truly, the movements they are responsible for can't meet the demands of our daily repetition. When we sit in poor postures or move in repetitious ways that don't support our alignment, stabilizers are less able to do their job of stabilizing our joints in a neutral position, and the involuntary, neurological mechanisms we rely on to move efficiently are altered. When it comes to shoulder or pelvic stabilizers, inhibited/ weak muscles tend to stay lengthened, adding to instability of the girdles in which they operate. Muscle movers then become chronically shortened, which can cause compression in joints, on nerves, and on vessels that supply vital blood flow to our extremities. This reduces grip strength and fine motor control of our hands, as well as stability and ground reaction control when we want to walk, run, or play sports.

We don't notice this decline in our shoulder or hip stability until our joints hurt when we move. This is how most people figure out that something is wrong—they don't know what it is specifically, but 90 percent of the time, this is what's causing pain in a joint during motion.

How the Two Rs of NeuroStrength Prevent This Inhibition

When you MELT and your connective tissue—the environment the sensory nerves live in—is properly hydrated, sensory motor control is more precise. This gives you more efficient neurological or sensorimotor control.

NeuroStrength focuses on reintegrating the timing of the deep stabilizers as a point of entry for recovering their function. By focusing on what's staying stable rather than the movement, you ultimately create a starting point to reopen the neurological potential for stabilization to occur.

When it comes to stability, timing is everything. The timing of stabilizing muscle contraction is initiated in the brain through neurons that create a complex motor signal. NeuroStrength restores the timing of the deep stabilizing mechanisms of your joints, particularly the pelvic and shoulder girdles.

Instead of building on a foundation of quicksand, getting exhausted by compensation, and unwittingly creating a stronger yet more dysfunctional body, for the very first time you can rebuild your foundation to improve neurological stability. This will allow you to keep reaching new goals in your training.

▶ The Development of NeuroStrength

I developed the Reintegration and Repatterning techniques when, during my hands-on work as a neuromuscular therapist, I used my skills to evaluate whether people were using proper muscular timing for movements. I was taught to identify when muscle timing was delayed, and I also learned how to use my hands to shut down poor patterns to reintegrate and repattern more efficient function. It took me years of practice on hundreds of clients to refine these skills.

The problem with these techniques, however, was that even though my evaluation and intervention restored my clients' neurological timing, I couldn't explain to them how to replicate my work at home to combat the new stress that would amass starting the moment they left my office. I could help them make changes in the right direction, but without their participation and awareness, it never lasted long. My clients' repetitive lifestyles and movement patterns would create new stuck stress, and so my clients would come back to me again and again for tune-ups.

So I began developing hands-off techniques that would simulate how I assessed and treated and reassessed each client. Since most people don't know the names of their muscles or even their bony landmarks, I spent time teaching my clients to set their body up in positions that would give them the best sense of what needed to remain stable before we executed the moves. Instead of talking anatomy, I explained exactly where and what they would feel if the neurological reintegrative process had kicked in or if they were relying on habitual compensatory pathways. This is often the most frustrating part of the process. Remember, every movement is a skill so when you start learning you'll have to think a lot to create these subtle movements. The upside is, over time, you'll have to think very little to move better and with less joint pain.

Reintegrate

The goal of Reintegration is to access and reacquire the neurological pathways of the deep stabilizing mechanisms so that proper timing of the appropriate muscles for core or girdle stabilization occurs before you move. Motor control depends not only on whether the brain's command is correct but whether the muscle can enact the command. For example, if you sit for eight hours a day, the deep stabilizers of your spine (muscles such as multifidus and psoas) can become impaired to contract at all.

In fact, muscles can undergo fundamental changes causing fibrosis or adipose (fat) accumulation. Even if you want to stand up and the brain sends a proper message, if muscles cannot pick up the impulse, your back will ache upon moving from seated to standing. Once the sensorimotor pathways are reopened, the body has the potential to maintain proper stabilization of the joints before and during movement in daily life. Not only do neurological pathways sustain pelvic and shoulder girdle stability, but reintegration involves muscles that leverage and stabilize the joints of our body as we move.

Although I can see whether integration is happening, my clients weren't watching themselves in a mirror to see its effect, so they had to learn to feel it—and you will too. If stabilization isn't integrated, it's easy for me to see instability once the body is in motion. Again, you have to learn what it *feels* like when your body is compensating or whether the mechanisms of stability have engaged to execute a MELT Performance move with skill. When neurological integration is present, the masses of the pelvis or torso remain stable in relatively the same position. If a compensatory pathway is used, the girdles move as you initiate any arm or leg movement. You won't feel the work in the right places; that's your cue to stop and start over. If you continue with more repetitions, you'll just be reinforcing the wrong pathways.

Since NeuroStrength is a self-treatment technique, your challenge for proper reintegration is the setup—how to position your body—and then knowing how to execute the move and identify what it feels like when you're doing it right or wrong.

Why Isn't the Concept of Reintegration Better Known?

The nervous system and sensorimotor control are not fundamental components of the fitness industry. Yet they should be. The fitness model of today has not changed significantly since the seventies: It's still focused on muscles—building them, toning them, strengthening them—and, to be honest, vanity. It's all about what you look like from the outside, not how you can function more efficiently and avoid pain and injuries.

Doing dozens of bicep curls does not necessarily improve joint stability, motor control, or posture. If neurologically, your brain can't produce proper sensorimotor control, you still do your bicep curls, but you compensate without knowing it, and you become a stronger, more dysfunctional person. You get better at managing your imbalances, but you don't really improve joint stability at all. It's actually what causes stress injuries.

Reintegration *is* about isolating movement, but not to improve muscle strength or size. Reintegration is about helping the brain receive and send information for more precise and efficient sensorimotor response.

What the fitness industry doesn't understand is that your joints are the areas of *detour.* They are the areas of accumulated stress that your body has to compensate for. This compensation starts a cascade of delayed or inhibited sensorimotor response. Compensation is what creates neurological inhibition, poor motor pathways, and structural imbalance. Although we will be working on activating certain motor pathways, I want you to remember: *It's not about the strength of a muscle; it's about the neurological stability pathways and mechanisms and how they activate.* Isolating a muscle to make it bigger or stronger just isn't the point of NeuroStrength.

According to traditional muscle theory, the agonist muscle is the primary mover and the antagonist muscle is what opposes the agonist. If you're doing a bicep curl, for example, the bicep is the agonist and the tricep on the other side of your upper arm is the antagonist. Here's the thing though: Fascia helps us manage movement so no muscle works in isolation. This means that traditional weightlifting doesn't address function—it merely adapts the shape and size of muscles.

When I started understanding neuromuscular therapy and how fascia leverages and disperses force laterally—not linearly through the muscle tendons—this very rudimentary muscle theory of agonist/antagonist that I had learned in college went right into the crapper. Dynamic human movement is not so mechanical. It's much more flow-y, and much more whole-body-induced. In fact, it has less to do with how strong you are and much more to do with how your motor pathways are able to remain open and connected to your sensory system so that the messages about how to move go back and forth efficiently. Through more recent research, we now understand that fascia disperses force laterally—not just along one muscle to contract so the opposing muscle relaxes, but to create a whole-body event in any motion so the rest of the body stays stable as we move or contract a muscle or move a joint. When fascia loses its supportive qualities from repetition or injury, motor timing to stabilize joints becomes faulty, yet we don't know this is happening because we are still moving. Just like the body builder with the shoulder pain doing a bench press—he recognized that the movement was the same, so what was different?

I realized that what gives your body strength and power is not the size of your muscles, but your neuromuscular control and stability. I came to understand that if your joints aren't stable, motor patterns become faulty. Why? Because your brain is trying to get around the detour of the unstable joint, to get any muscles to fire so you move the way you think you should. If it has to detour all the time, a cascade effect is set up, such as:

1. Fascia becomes too stiff and loses its supportive and adaptable qualities.

2. Muscle timing is altered.

3. Motor control and function become faulty.

4. You strain a tendon or ligament.

5. Joints misalign, become compressed or decentralized, or become hypermobile.

6. Muscles get inhibited or delayed in their contraction, or they get restricted and can't release with proper timing.

7. You strain more tendons and muscles.

8. You notice you walk with a limp, or your knee or hip or back hurt when you try to stand up and walk around, or you do the same Downward Dog pose, swing a golf club, or squat the same weight you've done a hundred times—and something pops, breaks, or snaps. And that's it. You are now injured.

You keep moving until you suddenly get to number eight on this list. You missed all of the pre-pain signals your body was sending well before you walked with a limp or were injured. Those are the sudden chronic pain symptoms. They seem to come on abruptly, but in fact stress has been accumulating and neurological stability has been faulty for a long time. But you haven't been taught to notice pre-pain signals.

Once you identify common imbalances and return connective tissue to its adaptable and supportive state, you are ready to reintegrate the timing and control of the deep stabilizing mechanisms. When fascia is hydrated, it's easier for you to rewire the proper pathways because the roadblocks are no longer there.

◗ Primary Principles of Reintegration

Reintegration is the first step to giving your body the NeuroStrength it needs to prevent faulty movements, sudden chronic pain, and repetitive stress injuries. The Reintegration *setup* is the secret to its success. The time you spend setting yourself up and getting your brain to remember the position is half the battle. Once you can put yourself into and remember the setup, a precise movement and pause occur. Once you reintegrate stability, repatterning is easy to achieve because it's essentially the same movement repeated at a different pace and sometimes with an increased range of motion.

There are three key principles of Reintegration:

1. PROPER SETUP AND POSITION ARE ESSENTIAL. The setup is the most important part of achieving neurological stability. You can't get sloppy with NeuroStrength moves. The position of your primary masses—the shoulder girdle, ribs/torso, and pelvis—is essential to reintegrate the neurological stabilization mechanisms. Sustaining the setup allows your primary pathways to ignite. Only when your primary masses are stable can you add repetitive motion to repattern the timing of your deep stabilizing muscles.

    You'll get detailed instructions about how to do the setups in Part Three, and the more you do them, the easier they become.

2. CONCENTRATE ON WHAT'S STAYING STABLE—NOT ON WHAT'S MOVING. Reintegrating stability is not about how big your range of motion is or your overall muscle strength. It's about activating the right neural pathways so the right muscles contract appropriately to create joint stabilization. You're doing this now slowly and thoughtfully so you can do it automatically later.

    The basic principle is this: Don't think about what's moving. Instead, think about what's staying stable before and as you move. The precision in each position is what's going to yield mega-results.

    Although you can use a mirror to help you see if your hips or shoulder girdle are remaining where you want them, you might visually miss your own compensation. You have to learn to feel your own ability to stay stable. When you do the setup and execute the movement correctly, the masses of your pelvis, ribs, and shoulders have to remain still. If you reintegrate the right pathway, you'll feel the fatigue and work of these deep stabilizers rather quickly.

If you're not feeling it in the right place, most likely your setup position changed the moment you moved. You'll reset and check your setup at least twice during the Reintegration and Repatterning sets!

3. **TIMING IS EVERYTHING.** The final factor in the Reintegration process is timing. Once you find the proper pathway, you need to pause without compensation so your body can reintegrate this pathway.

   After the initial pause, Reintegration requires slow movement, a small range of motion, and another pause at the end range. Then with the same pace you'll slowly return to the beginning position without releasing the muscles. Again you'll pause and repeat the movement a total of only four times. That's it! This is where reintegration occurs. You have only four chances to reintegrate the proper pathway, then you need to move on. (You can always try again later.) Don't rush through any motion, as you will defeat the purpose and results. Spend the time needed to set up the correct position and execute a precise, small range of motion.

   When we do the NeuroStrength moves, I'll give you what I call multitask cues, to keep you focused on reintegration and away from compensation.

▶ Repattern

After one of my MELT classes, a strong, vibrant man in his twenties sought me out. He was lean and fit; he worked out five or six days a week and enjoyed participating in regular triathlons. Yet, he was in terrible pain. Why? Because all of the accumulated stress he'd amassed while doing his training and then sitting at his desk working for eight hours every day caused compensatory patterns. He built strength on an unstable foundation, and on a structural level, he was "stuck in a tuck." His low back was paying the price for hip stabilizers that were very out of balance from the powerful muscle movers he had overtrained on many levels. He was unknowingly bracing his body by tucking his pelvis under and squeezing his butt because his back was so tight, leaving his whole structure completely out of balance. He told me that his favorite workout was to ride his bike for miles and then go for a run, and that afterward, his back killed him. I asked him what he did after these strenuous morning training routines.

"I go to work," he said.

"Do you stretch or do any basic stability work?" I asked.

"Not really. I heard that stretching muscles makes them weak, so I don't stretch much. But sometimes I do laps in the pool instead of a run," he replied, like that was the alternative to stretching and doing stability work.

"That's not a replacement for stability or restoring efficiency. I get that you think the more you train, the stronger and better you'll become at those activities, but it seems to me you're training yourself into dysfunction."

We agreed to test his hip stability so that I could show him that even though he thought his hips were strong, they were actually unstable. So I set him up to do a proper Side Leg Lift to test his lateral hip stabilizers. He couldn't lift his leg at all unless he cheated and moved his hip to make it look like he was lifting his leg.

"I don't get it," he said. "If I can ride a bike for miles and run a marathon, how come I can't lift my leg out to the side? That doesn't make any sense."

I explained to him that you can be as strong as an ox on a structural level, yet be in a chronic state of compensation on a neurological level because of repetitive movement. Often when I muscle test a body builder with hip pain using this NeuroStrength move, they lean forward and use their obliques, thus their pelvis acts like a hinge because they literally can't isolate movement in abduction at the hip joint. Their muscle movers overtake the range of motion, and the compensation is so profound that they often have less neurological stability than someone who's never set foot inside a gym. How did they get this way? Body builders are brilliant at repetitive, seemingly isolated motion. That's what weight lifting is. They do the same isolated moves over and over, bulking up the shape of their muscles without realizing the damage they're doing to the neurological stability of their joints.

I see this phenomenon happen all the time—not just to body builders, of course, but to people who think their workouts do nothing but good for their bodies. Such as yogis. Yoga is a terrific discipline that can do wonders for your strength, flexibility, breath control, and state of mind—when it's done right. I've had many, many yoga teachers and practitioners—who were, obviously, expert at yoga poses—still have tendon and ligament strains and sprains and joint damage. I always explain to them that when I used to lift weights, my form was so impeccable that people would watch me in the gym to learn what to do. The body builders who had been my teachers taught me precision and form, to slow down, to control each move, to do twelve repetitions, and then to increase the weight. If I started getting sloppy, I stopped; it was always better to do four perfect reps than eight sloppy ones. That was my weight-lifting foundation. I assumed that because my form was so good, my foundation was, too—but it was actually faulty from day one because I didn't yet have any real understanding of neurological stability, and the guys in the gym who were generous enough to teach me didn't have it either.

This is why so many yogis and dancers get repetitive stress injuries. They are strong but segmentally flexible in some regions, super tight in others, and hypermobile around their joints.

What you need, and what all of these hurting and injured fitness enthusiasts and professionals need, is to use the principles of MELT Performance to change the way you move by restoring neurological stability. By executing Reintegration, you are restoring stability of the joints and then repatterning movement with that newfound stability. This is the recipe for a pain-free, active lifestyle for years to come.

▶ Restoring Primary Movement Patterns

Neuroscientists used to believe that once you laid the neurological pathways (for language, movement, or other functions) when you were young, that was it. We now know that you can alter movement behavior and rewire your neuronal pathways at any age. Think of repatterning movement as a way to help your brain create new neural connections.

Repatterning is all about restoring functional patterns through muscular timing and joint stabilization. It is always done *after* you Reintegrate. The goal of repatterning is to restore proper, efficient motor patterns by applying a basic movement to a reintegrated pathway. Once you activate a proper stability pathway, you can improve your natural, primal patterns and reacquire or restore efficient motion of your arms or legs. As a result, day-to-day movement is more effortlessly achieved without compensation and you'll be moving the way you're supposed to be moving! The more stable your body is, the more coordinated you'll be.

Remember, the Reintegration sets allow these stabilizing muscles time to properly activate. If you are compensating during Reintegration, you'll have to reset your setup position many times or you'll feel the work in the wrong places. If you notice these things, you aren't ready to repattern the movement. I know this may get frustrating, especially if you're used to muscling your way through life and pushing through pain and fatigue, but you haven't yet found the neurological pathway you want to reinforce with Repatterning.

However, once you do find the proper pathways and are able to sense your own stability, you can hardwire the proper timing between stabilizers and movers with Repattern techniques, thus reducing your risk of injuring a shoulder, hip, or knee or having low back or neck pain. In fact, once proper neurological connection has been adopted and stability has been reacquired, you'll notice you move more freely and your overall energy is more resilient.

▶ Primary Principles of Repatterning

After you reintegrate the proper neurological pathway, you're ready to repattern movement. There are three key principles of Repatterning:

1. CONCENTRATE ON WHAT'S STAYING STABLE—NOT ON WHAT'S MOVING. Here it is again. Just like Reintegration needs the focus to be on the masses remaining stable as you move your arms or legs, this concept is even more critical because now you're going to move through a larger range of motion. Your brain is going to want to take over and divert you back on the side street. This is again like a Jedi mind trick: You've got to use your Body Sense; focus even more on the stability before mobility. Don't rush through the range of motion. Really draw your attention to maintaining contact with your core and then execute the four repetitions as smoothly and with as much control as you can.

2. THERE'S NO PAUSING AS YOU MOVE FROM ONE POINT TO THE NEXT. Once you properly set up your body position during Reintegration, and then challenge the stabilizing mechanism to function with accuracy, fatigue sets in quickly if you've reintegrated the proper pathways. Remember, you'll do only four repetitions in a Reintegration set. Then, you want to hardwire the actual sensorimotor pathway. To do this, you'll increase the range of motion and lose the pause at the end range to coordinate a basic, primal pattern. Make sure you are feeling the work in the right place before you do a Repattern set. Repattern sets should be slow, smooth, and controlled, but the pace is slightly faster than the Reintegration sets. When you create a pattern, consistent movement is necessary. Think of it

like walking. You don't pause for a second every time your foot hits the ground. Movement is seamless and dynamic when a body is stable. So engaging the pattern means moving smoothly, consistently, and slowly through the full range of motion you're trying to restore.

3. **FOUR IS THE MAGIC NUMBER.** Four repetitions to reintegrate a stability pathway, and four repetitions to lock in the pattern is all it takes to begin improving sensorimotor control if done properly. Doing more repetitions won't reinforce a newfound pathway. Remember, your body is designed to compensate and find the path of least resistance, which is the wrong pathway and not the one you want to reinforce.

Now that you understand the basic concepts of Reintegration and Repatterning, let's put this theory into motion with the Side Leg Lift.

Side Leg Lift

SETUP

1. *Lie comfortably on your side with your head on your arm, or use a pillow to support your neck. Bend your bottom knee at 90 degrees. You want to feel that you're lying on your outer thigh rather than on your hip bone. Shift your hips back if you feel like you're lying uncomfortably on your hip bone. Place your ankle joint on top of the roller.*

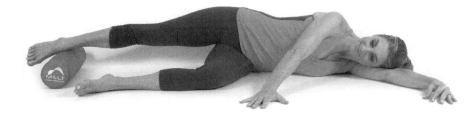

2. *Tilt, Stack, and Roll (see page 215) with your top hand on your hip, and find your core.*

REINTEGRATE SET 1

1. *Keep your pelvis stable and slowly lift your top leg so that it's parallel to the floor. Keep your leg in line with your torso; avoid flexing the hip joint. Reset your Tilt, Stack, and Roll with your leg remaining lifted and hold this position for 10 to 15 seconds. Place your top hand on the floor to stabilize your torso, and find your core.*

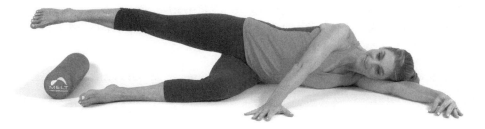

2. *Now internally rotate your leg and pause for 2 counts, then externally rotate your leg from your hip joint, keeping your pelvis stable, and pause for 2 counts. Repeat this rotation 4 times, focusing on keeping your pelvis still and in the Tilt, Stack, and Roll position.*

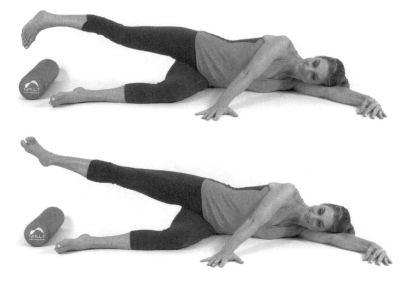

REINTEGRATE SET 2

1. *Recheck your pelvic position, keep your thigh slightly internally rotated, and then lift your leg 1 inch higher and pause for 2 counts. Lower your thigh so it's parallel to the floor and pause for 2 counts.*

2. *Repeat this small range of motion 4 times, pausing at the top range and at parallel during each repetition.*

REPATTERN SET 1

1. *Recheck your Tilt, Stack, and Roll. Slowly lift the leg again to your top range without your pelvis moving at all, and then lower it until your ankle hits the roller but don't relax.*

2. *Slowly and smoothly lift again through the full range, with no pause, 4 times.*

REPATTERN SET 2

1. *Lift your leg to your end range, about 1 inch higher than parallel to the floor, with your pelvis remaining in the optimal position, and create internal-to-external rotation of the leg 4 times as you did in Reintegrate, only this time without pausing. (Internal rotation is done by turning your thigh inward to face the floor; external rotation moves the front thigh toward the ceiling with no pelvic motion.)*

Rest Reassess

1. *Scan your masses and spaces and notice whether any imbalances are decreased.*

2. *Are your ribs, pelvis, and thighs more relaxed on the floor? Is your low back less tense and arched? Can you turn your head more efficiently?*

3. *Does your Autopilot have a clear connection to your center of gravity?*

    – *Do you feel more even from left to right?*

4. *Notice and remember what you feel.*

The Side Leg Lift you do in MELT Performance might have the same name as the Jane Fonda exercise, but it couldn't be more different. You'll only do four repetitions of rotation and four repetitions lifting and lowering your leg in a very small range to reintegrate the timing of the side hip stabilizers. You'll then do the same amount of repetitions when you repattern but increase the range and lose the pause between repetitions. If you think you can do more repetitions, I'm sorry to tell you but you're using the wrong pathway and you aren't improving stability at all. Stabilizing mechanisms fatigue quickly, so when you utilize them and access them without compensation, you'll know it.

In fact, in the first video we did for MELT Performance, my friend and colleague Gregg Cook, who's an accomplished fitness professional with the body of an Adonis, struggled to do my Side Leg Lift at first. He couldn't believe how hard it was to sustain the proper position and execute such small and simple moves. Even strong bodies have issues with stability, so don't be fooled. Once you slow down and focus on what's staying stable, and then you do the very precise, very slow movements, you will rewire your neurological pathways—and you'll be on your way to improved performance. You'll find over a short period of time that you'll acquire better control and execute the movements with greater ease. But I have to let you know: These moves will never be easy! (If they are, you're doing them wrong!) Again, stabilizing muscles don't like to work independently of muscle movers; quite frankly, muscle movers most often are trying to stabilize a joint because the true stabilizers are inhibited to engage in the first place. But if a muscle mover is doing an extra job of stabilization, when you try to move, it's already busy doing something else. So your movements become less accurate and your joints pay the price.

7

NeuroStrength Moves

A s you know by now, awareness and focus are essential to improving your NeuroStrength. Just as important as the Rest Assess and Rest Reassess are to helping you improve Body Sense and building your self-awareness, the setup of each move is the most important element to truly reintegrating the timing of your stabilizing potential.

You'll know when you properly reintegrate the correct stabilizing pathways by where you feel the work occurring. For example, when you do the Side Lying Arm Fans, ensuring that your elbow stays in front of your hip and that you sense the work on the side of your shoulder is specifically what you want to focus on and feel. If you set up your position and feel strain or work in your neck or forearm, your body is telling you that it's still using the wrong pathway to stabilize the shoulder in that position. Your best bet is to stop and try to reset your body position. If you still feel that your body can't reintegrate stability, don't get frustrated. Instead, turn over and start on your other side.

Often, we can reintegrate stabilization on one side of the body more quickly and accurately than on the other. However, when you turn back over, you should have an internal conversation with your body and "ask" it to find the same position and connection as you just did on the other side. You might be surprised to find that your conscious encouragement and focus can reset the stabilization mechanisms right in that very moment. If you have faulty pathways, your body only knows how to move in the path of least resistance. If compensation has been present for many years, it may take you a few tries to achieve the results I want you to obtain. Be patient and give your neural pathways some time to repave a new highway to stability.

If you find that a move is difficult or you can't acquire reintegration, try another move and see whether you can reintegrate the stabilizing mechanisms. For example, if Side Lying Arm Fans is challenging the first few times, move on to Side Lying Backhand and see whether you can reintegrate the timing of that stability pathway and then return to Side Lying Arm Fans to try again with greater success.

Be patient with your body and give the reintegration process time. Your body is designed to adapt, but sometimes it takes a little extra focus and time to reset a body baseline. You can do this!

When you use the resistance band with the upper body moves, setting up the band and how you initially grab it are essential. You need to use the same amount of resistance on each side. Try to set up the position in the same way each time you try the move. You can also use a pillow under your head for more comfort when you do any of these side lying moves.

Remember, to reintegrate the stability pathways the setup is the key factor. To repattern sensorimotor control, you must focus on what's staying stable as you move. Don't muscle your way through the set or increase your pace as compensatory pathways are ready to take over at any moment.

▶ Upper Body Stability Moves

Side Lying Arm Fans

This move reintegrates the deep stabilizers of your shoulder called the rotator cuff. External rotation is the movement you are going to ultimately repattern. These stabilizers are often inhibited and weak.

    Note: If you sense strain or pain in your neck or forearm, stop and return to the setup, or flip over and try it on your other arm first.

SETUP

1. *Place the resistance band on the floor and lie comfortably on your left side with the band underneath your hip to keep the band in place.*

2. *Reach your bottom arm out from under you so you're lying more on your ribs and outer shoulder blade, not on your shoulder joint or arm.*

3. *Send your bottom hip back so you're lying more on the side of your thigh than your outer hip bone. Bend both knees at approximately 45 degrees.*

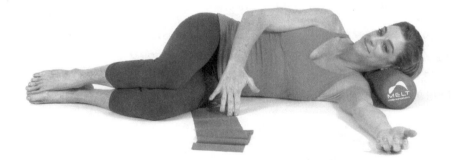

4. Practice the range of motion first without the band. Internally and externally rotate your shoulder joint while keeping your elbow touching the front of your hip bone. Don't let your elbow float behind you as you externally rotate your shoulder joint.

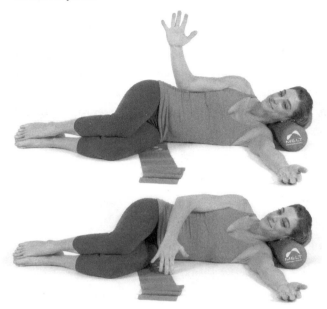

5. Keep your elbow in front of your hip bone and reach to the floor to grab the band. Crumple up the band to create a handle to hold on to.

6. Pull up on the band and return your forearm to being parallel to the floor, keeping your wrist and hand in line with your arm. You should now feel moderate tension on the band as you hold this position for 10 to 15 seconds to initiate the reintegration process.

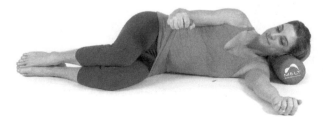

REINTEGRATE SET 1

1. *Slowly punch your arm forward to increase tension on the band (angle the punch ahead of your hip, rather than your shoulder), pause for 2 counts, and then slowly bend the elbow, letting it pass your hip, keeping the forearm parallel to the floor and tension on the band. Your hand should float over your hip. Repeat this movement 4 times, pausing with your arm extended in front of your hip for 2 counts with tension on the band.*

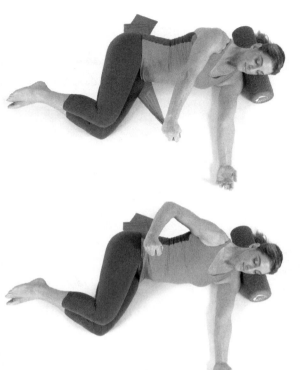

2. *Repeat this move 3 to 4 times to reintegrate the shoulder stabilizers and override the muscle movers (your anterior deltoid). On your last move, slow down and stop before your elbow passes your hip.*

3. *Hold the position—the elbow bent just in front of the hip but not resting on it—for 10 to 15 seconds. If you need to, you can place your index finger or your fist under your elbow joint to assist in holding your arm in the proper position.*

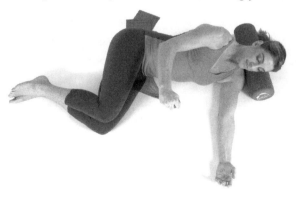

1. *Keep your opposite fist or finger under your elbow to help maintain proper form during this set if necessary.*

2. *Pull up on the band and increase its tension, so that your forearm angles upward, toward where the ceiling meets the wall in front of you while keeping your elbow stationary for 4 counts; then pause for 2 counts.*

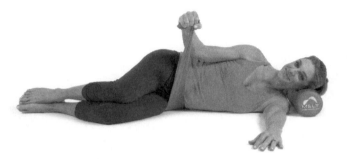

3. *Return your forearm to parallel for 4 counts and then pause in this position for 2 counts.*

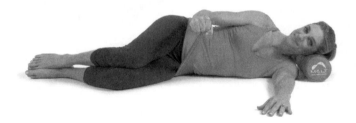

4. *Repeat 4 times while multitasking.*

MULTITASK: *Your elbow stays in front of the body as you externally rotate your arm from your shoulder joint, ear away from the shoulder, no shrugging, wrist in line with the forearm. Avoid extending your wrist as you externally rotate your shoulder joint.*

Note: *Like a Jedi, you must continue to distract the mind from the movement. Multitasking is necessary. Constantly tuning into your set up position and precision of what's staying stable as you move is part of the multitasking process. I want you thinking of these things as you move. This can be somewhat exhausting to the brain but that's part of what reintegrates a new neural pathway instead of allowing your body to be satisfied with your movement outcome.*

REPATTERN SET 1

1. *In the same range of motion, increase your pace slightly and don't pause at the end range to reintegrate the timing of your external shoulder rotators. Repeat this motion 4 times.*

Note: *Remove your finger or fist from under your elbow unless needed for proper form.*

REPATTERN SET 2

1. *Drop the band and repeat the motion 4 times while multitasking. Try to increase the range of motion.*

2. *Repeat on the other arm.*

You want to feel

+ *Fatigue or burning in the shoulder joint and rear upper arm*

Stop immediately if you feel

− *Strain or pain in the neck, collarbones, forearms, biceps, or wrists*

MELT Prep Sequence Helpers

▶ *Do any or all of these sequences first to prepare your body for Side Lying Arm Fans: Performance Hand Treatment (page 131), Upper Body Rehydrate Sequence (page 145), Neck Release Sequence (page 176).*

▶ *If you have trouble with this move, try Side Lying Backhand (page 210).*

Common Compensations

If your shoulder girdle is unstable, your elbow will travel behind the body, your shoulder blade will move toward your spine, your wrist will extend, or your forearm will rotate.

Side Lying Backhand

This move reintegrates the rear or posterior shoulder stabilizer called the rear deltoid. Lateral extension is the movement you are going to reacquire. These stabilizers are often inhibited and weak.

Note: *If you sense strain or pain in your neck or forearm, stop and return to the setup or flip over and try the move on your other arm first.*

Using imagery for this move will give you a better sense of the range of motion. Think about trying to pull up a bucket of water without it tipping over, so the range of motion remains in front of your body at all times.

SETUP

1. *Like Side Lying Arm Fans, lie on your left side with the band underneath your hip.*

2. *Reach your bottom arm out from under you so you're lying more on your ribs and outer shoulder blade, not on your shoulder joint or arm.*

3. *Send your bottom hip back so you're lying more on the side of your thigh than on your outer hip bone. Bend both knees at approximately 45 degrees.*

4. *Raise your right arm toward the ceiling. Notice how your shoulder and arm naturally feel on top of one another. Move your shoulder away from your ear, and allow your arm to angle a little so that your hand is over your hip, rather than over your shoulder.*

5. *Keep your arm straight and lower it toward and away from the floor 4 times. Sense what it feels like for the shoulder to be heavy in the socket.*

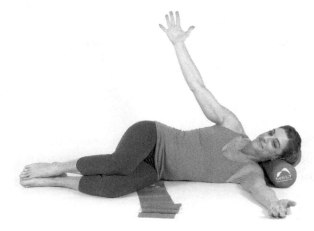

6. Sink your shoulder into the socket and keep your torso completely still as you lower your arm down to the floor and grab the band at the length of your arm. Crumple up the band to make a loose handle.

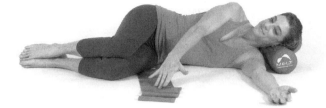

REINTEGRATE SET 1

1. Keep your wrist in line with your forearm (don't flex or extend the wrist) as you pull your arm up so it's parallel to the floor. You should feel moderate tension on the band. The hand should look as if it's in front of the hip. Hold this position for 10 seconds to initiate the reintegration process.

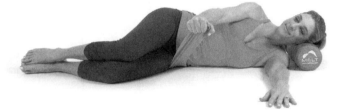

2. As you did with Side Lying Arm Fans, slowly punch your arm forward in front of your hip joint (rather than your shoulder) to increase tension on the band, pause for 2 counts, and then slowly bend the elbow, letting it pass your hip, keeping the forearm parallel to the floor and tension on the band. Your hand should float over your hip. Repeat this movement 4 times, pausing at the end range for 2 counts with tension consistently on the band.

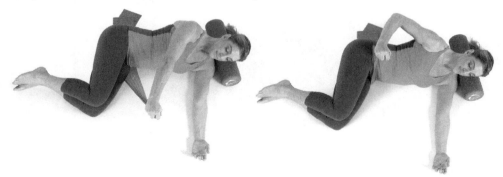

3. *End with your arm extended in front of your hip, parallel to the floor, for 10 to 15 seconds.*

REINTEGRATE SET 2

1. *Keep tension on the band and slowly raise your arm for 4 counts. Imagine that the pinky side of your arm is leading the motion without rotating the forearm, palm stays facedown. Stop when your hand points toward where the ceiling meets the wall, and pause for 2 counts.*

2. *Slowly lower your arm back to parallel for 4 counts. Notice how the band remains taut through the range of motion. Hold this position for a breath and wait for 2 counts.*

   - *Your arm should be in line with your hip and not angled toward your shoulder.*

   - *The motion of the arm is up rather than back—as if you're lifting a bucket of water.*

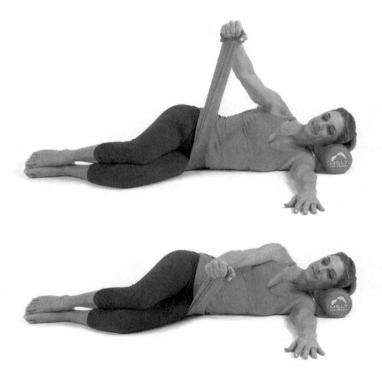

3. Slowly repeat this motion 4 times. Pause at the top range for 2 counts, and then slowly lower your arm back to parallel for 4 counts. If you place your opposite hand over the front of your shoulder joint to increase awareness of what's moving your arm, you shouldn't feel your torso move as the arm moves.

4. Repeat this range of motion 4 times while multitasking.

MULTITASK: *The movement occurs between the arm and shoulder blade, not between the shoulder blade and the spine. Your wrist stays in line with your forearm, your shoulder away from your ear, no shrugging, and your torso is stable. Don't hyperextend your elbow. Your arm remains angled between your shoulder and hip. Your core remains active.*

REPATTERN SET 1

1. Slowly lift and lower the arm, without pausing, 4 times with the same range of motion while multitasking.

REPATTERN SET 2

1. Drop the band and increase the motion to your full range, without moving your torso, 4 times while multitasking.

2. Repeat on the other arm.

You want to feel

+ Fatigue or burning in the back and side of the shoulder joint and rear upper arm

Stop immediately if you feel

− Strain or pain in the neck, collarbones, forearms, biceps, or wrists

− That it's easy or you can't sense any shoulder work

− More work in your arm than in your shoulder

MELT Prep Sequence Helpers

▶ *Do these first to prepare your body for Side Lying Backhand: Performance Hand Treatment (page 131), Upper Body Rehydrate Sequence (page 145), and Neck Release Sequence (page 176).*

▶ *If you can't do Side Lying Backhand, try Side Lying Arm Fans (page 205).*

Common Compensations

You may find you rotate your torso, have your arm in line with your shoulder or face, or lock out or hyperextend your elbow. You may also notice you shrug your shoulder toward your ear or lean back to let your muscle movers between the shoulder girdle and the spine do the work.

▶ Lower Body Stability Moves

Tilt, Stack, and Roll

Before you try to reintegrate the stability pathways of your pelvis, you need to set up the proper pelvic position. For all three lower body stability moves, the tilt that you've already practiced is an important part of the setup. To reduce compensation when you're lying on your side, you'll also have to actively stack your top hip on top of the bottom hip.

Both the Clam and Side Leg Lift require one more subtle addition: As you lift your leg in either move, your top hip will want to roll backward. So for these two moves, you'll need to roll your top hip forward slightly to minimize this common compensation.

Let's practice all three components of this important pelvic position:

1. **TILT** *your pelvis slightly so your low back has a natural curve. Your ribs remain neutral. Don't jut your chest out to tilt.*

2. **STACK** *your hips by placing your top hand on the top of your hip bone and reaching or pushing it away from your ribs. Sense this as increased space in your waistline. Make sure your ribs stay relaxed on the floor.*

3. **ROLL** *your top hip forward so your upper knee bypasses your lower knee by one inch. Your ribs stay heavy and relaxed. Your top knee is now slightly in front of your bottom knee.*

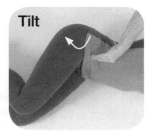
Tilt

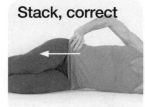
Stack, correct

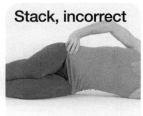
Stack, incorrect

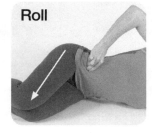
Roll

Clams

This move reintegrates the timing of the external hip rotators such as the piriformis, obturator internus and externus, gemellus inferior and superior, and quadratus femoris. These stabilizers are often inhibited and weak, so they don't provide essential control for movements like running and jumping. Improving the timing of these stabilizers mitigates the risk of patella-femoral and anterior cruciate ligament (ACL) injuries and improves rotational power—an essential advantage to athleticism.

Note: *If you sense low back strain or work in the hip resting on the floor, stop and reset. These are signs of compensation.*

This is a great move for people who have SI pain, knee and hamstring issues, and foot pain.

SETUP

1. *Lie on your side and rest your head on the roller.*

2. *Reach your bottom arm slightly forward so you're not lying on your shoulder joint. Relax your arm.*

3. *Bend both knees at approximately 45 degrees. Your heels should be in line with your sits bones. Your hips should be in line with your shoulders, and the outer part of your bottom foot should rest on the floor.*

4. *Send your bottom hip back so you aren't lying on your hip bone. You want to feel like you are lying on your outer thigh.*

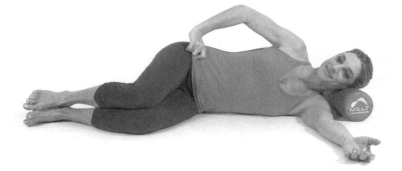

5. *Tilt, Stack, and Roll: Tilt your pelvis slightly so your low back has a natural curve. Your ribs remain neutral. Don't jut your chest out to tilt. Stack your hips by placing*

your hand on your top pelvic bone and reaching or pushing it away from your top ribs to increase space in the waistline. Sense this increased space in your waistline away from the floor, but don't let your ribs lift. Roll your top hip forward so your upper knee bypasses your lower knee by 1 inch. Your ribs stay heavy and relaxed. Your top knee is now slightly in front of your bottom knee.

6. *Find your core using your 3-D Breath to sustain the setup position.*

REINTEGRATE SET 1

1. *Keep your heels together and slowly externally rotate your top leg into the clam position. Think of reaching your top knee forward as you lift your top leg without moving your pelvis or torso backward, then pause.*

2. *As you hold this position for 10 to 15 seconds, your Autopilot will try to compensate and readjust your setup position without your conscious awareness. Eliminate this natural compensation by resetting the Tilt, Stack, and Roll, only this time with your leg in the clam position.*

3. *Keep your heels pressed together (your toes can be apart), and try to lift your leg slightly more into external rotation.*

4. *As you hold this position, make sure that proper reintegration is occurring: Put your top hand on the floor in front of you with your elbow extended. Slowly try to decompress the weight of your lower thigh from the floor. This is a very subtle movement. (You don't need to lift the leg off the floor. The objective is to reduce the compensation of pressing your lower thigh into the floor to hold the upper leg's position.) Hold this slight decompression of the lower leg for 5 to 10 seconds while keeping your top thigh in the clam position.*

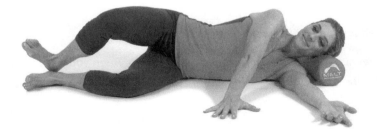

5. *Return your lower leg to the floor as you try to clam the top leg a little farther without moving your hips backward.*

6. *Hold this for 5 seconds to initiate better integration in the top hip. In total, you have held this position, reset, and increased range for approximately 30 seconds.*

REINTEGRATE SET 2

1. *Slowly lower your top leg back to the lower leg. Note that your top knee should still be in front of the lower knee.*

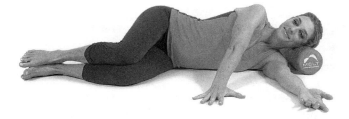

2. *Slowly lift the top thigh up again into external rotation at the hip for 4 counts, pause, and hold at that end range for 4 counts. Then slowly return your top leg down to the bottom leg for 4 counts with your upper knee still in front of the bottom knee. Keep your hips from moving forward or backward through the range. Think about reaching your top knee forward as you lift.*

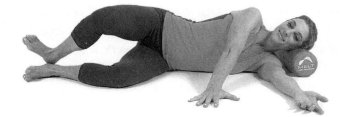

3. *Check your Tilt, Stack, and Roll position.*

4. *Repeat 4 times pausing at the end range while multitasking. Keep your hips stable throughout the full range and with all four repetitions.*

MULTITASK: *Sustain and check your Tilt, Stack, and Roll setup position. Keep your top knee in front of the bottom knee at all times. Your ribs stay back and out of the movement.*

REPATTERN SET 1

1. *Lift and lower 4 times without pausing or relaxing through the full range of motion while multitasking.*

You want to feel

+ *Fatigue or work in the lower region of the hip where your leg meets the pelvis*

Stop immediately if you feel

− *Fatigue or work in the front thigh or down the leg, or the bottom hip (on the floor)*

− *Pain or strain in the low back, waist region, shoulders, or neck*

MELT Prep Sequence Helpers

▶ *Do these first to prepare your body for Clams: Seated Compression Sequence (page 170), Lower Body Rehydrate and Low Back Release Sequence (page 159), and Performance Foot Treatment (page 136).*

▶ *If you have a hard time reintegrating the deep hip with Clams, try Mini Bridge (page 229) or Side Leg Lift (page 199).*

Common Compensations

When your external hip rotators are not firing properly, the common compensation is for your pelvis to roll back as you lift the top leg into external rotation, recruiting low back stabilizers rather than hip joint stabilizers to initiate the movement. Your hips will not remain stacked, and your pelvis will tuck under. Another compensation is to press your bottom leg into the ground.

Inner Thigh Lift

The hip adductors are part of our Rooted Core and assist us in everything from standing to walking, and to moving quickly left to right. Their timing is essential to reduce hip and knee pain as well as accidental falls and ankle sprains.

For those who have low back or knee issues, incontinence, neck pain, or postpartum pain or who have had a C-section, this is an essential move to perfect.

SETUP

1. *Lie on your side with the roller in front of you.*

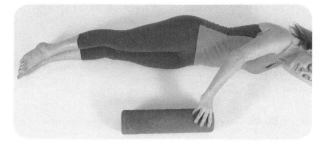

2. *Bend your top knee and place your lower leg on the top of the roller, from your knee to the inner arch of your foot. Your foot needs to remain elevated from the floor and not touching the ground. Adjust the position of the roller if necessary. Keep your bottom leg straight.*

   – *Don't roll forward to place your shin on the roller. Remain in a perfect side lying position for the proper setup.*

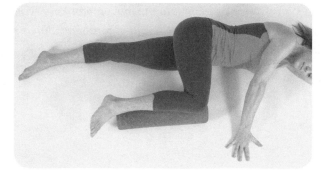

3. Place your top hand on your hip bone and set your pelvis into a slight tilt. Keep your ribs stable.

4. Stack your top hip on top of the bottom hip. Your waistline should lift slightly, but your ribs should remain heavy on the floor. Don't exaggerate the movement.

5. Find your core using your 3-D Breath.

REINTEGRATE SET 1

1. Move your top hand to your waistline to sense whether you feel muscle activation above your pelvis as you raise your bottom leg off the floor.

2. If you feel muscles at your waistline engage, set your leg down, roll your top hip backward just an inch, keep your pelvis tilted and stacked, find your core, slow down, and lift the bottom leg off the floor again. Energize your bottom heel away from your bottom hip but don't lose the stack of your hips.

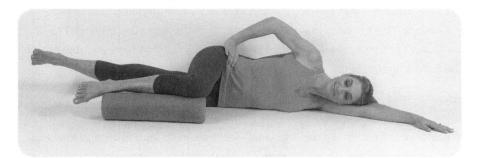

3. Sustain this lifted position and slowly move the bottom leg toward the roller by slightly flexing at your hip, and then lift the leg a little higher without moving your upper hip toward your ribs.

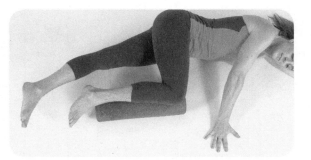

4. *Hold this position for 30 seconds. To check that the inner thigh is working properly, put your top hand on the floor, and without fully lifting your shin, think about decompressing the weight of the shin from the roller for 4 seconds. (You don't have to physically elevate the shin from the roller; just try lightening the weight of your shin to minimize compensation.) Slowly allow your upper shin to gently rest back on top of the roller to prepare for Set 2.*

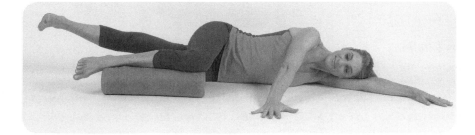

REINTEGRATE SET 2

1. *With your bottom leg still lifted, try to lift the leg a few inches higher, pause for 2 counts, and lower to the original position (not resting on the floor!) for 2 counts, and pause again. Make sure you pause both at the high and low range each time without releasing or relaxing at either point.*

2. *Repeat 4 times while multitasking.*

MULTITASK: *Your bottom leg reaches away from your hip as you lift and lower the leg. Your waist stays long and your core engaged. Check that the inner arch of your foot remains parallel to the floor. Don't sickle or curl your ankle inward (inversion of the foot) or rotate your toes upward (internal rotation of the hip).*

Note: *This move can be small. It's about reintegrating connection and control, not the movement or range of motion.*

REPATTERN SET 1

1. *Slowly and smoothly lift the leg to your end range.*

2. *Slowly lower your leg down to the floor without releasing the contraction or relaxing at all, and then lift the leg back up at the same pace. Don't pause at either point.*

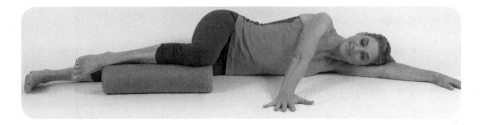

3. *Repeat 4 times while multitasking.*

REPATTERN SET 2

1. *Pause and hold at the top of the lift, check your setup, and make a slow, controlled, small 1 count pulse up and 1 count pulse down just an inch 4 times.*

2. *Hold at the top for 5 seconds and then release fully.*

You want to feel

+ *Fatigue or work in the inner thigh, closer to the hip*

Stop immediately if you feel

− *Pain or strain in the knee or low back*

MELT Prep Sequence Helpers

▶ *Do any of these sequences to prepare your body for Inner Thigh Lift: Lower Body Rehydrate and Low Back Release Sequence (page 159), Seated Compression Sequence (page 170), or Performance Foot Treatment (page 136).*

▶ *If you can't do Inner Thigh Lift, try Mini Bridge (page 229) or the Core Challenge (page 233).*

Common Compensations

When the adductors are not firing properly, the external obliques and quadratus lumborum (muscle above your waistline that acts upon pelvic motion) often get involved as the initiators of the move. Keep your hand on your waist and make sure that this compensation doesn't occur and your pelvis doesn't move from the setup position.

Side Leg Lift

You practiced this move in Chapter 6. It's especially crucial because an important role of the hip abductors is to stabilize your pelvis when you walk. When these stabilizers are inhibited, your walking gait and your overall balance can be affected. This can lead to low back pain and alter your NeuroCore control. A key low back and pelvic stabilizer, the quadratus lumborum, can get overactive to compensate for hip instability, causing further low back and neck compression and pain.

This is a great move for people who have low back or knee issues, SI pain, or foot pain.

SETUP

1. Lie on your side and rest your head on your arm or a pillow. Bend your bottom leg at a 90-degree angle. Remember, you want to feel like you're lying on the side of your thigh, not your hip bone, so if you need to, set your top foot on the ground and push your bottom hip back so you're lying on your outer thigh rather than your hip. Then reset your top leg straight so your ankle, knee, hip, shoulder, and ear are all lined up, and your inner ankle is resting on the roller.

2. Tilt, Stack, and Roll: Tilt your pelvis without moving your ribs forward. Stack your hips by placing your hand on your top hip and reaching your top leg away so your lower waistline feels like it has lifted off the floor slightly without your ribs moving. Roll your top hip forward slightly to help sustain the proper pelvic position.

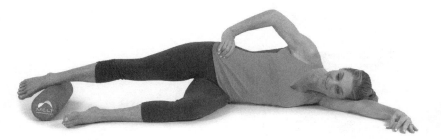

3. Find your core by using your 3-D Breath.

1. *Lift your leg off the roller so it's parallel to the floor. Reset your Tilt, Stack, and Roll while keeping your core engaged. Hold for 10 to 15 seconds. Place your top hand on the floor to stabilize your torso and find your core.*

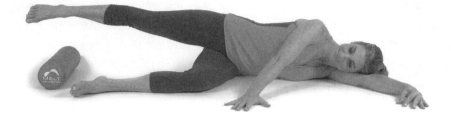

2. *Keep your pelvis stable. With the leg parallel to the floor, rotate the leg in so your toes point downward, pause (hold 2 counts), return to center, pause (hold 2 counts), externally rotate your thigh so your toes point upward, pause (hold 2 counts), then return back to center, pause (hold 2 counts)—all without moving your pelvis or torso. Repeat the rotation 4 times, pausing for 2 counts at each position while multitasking. End with an internal rotation. Be sure to rotate the whole leg and not just the lower leg.*

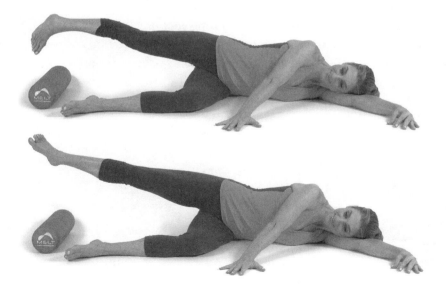

REINTEGRATE SET 2

1. *Keeping your leg internally rotated, slowly raise the leg a few inches higher and pause for 2 counts. Then lower your leg slowly just to parallel to the floor and pause again for 2 counts.*

2. *Slowly lower your leg back to parallel for 2 counts and pause for 2 counts.*

3. *Repeat 4 times while multitasking.*

MULTITASK: *Maintain your Tilt, Stack, and Roll and sustain your core contact. Return your hand to your pelvis at any point to build awareness of pelvic motion during Reintegration or to help sustain proper form.*

REPATTERN SET 1

1. *Recheck your Tilt, Stack, and Roll while keeping your core engaged.*

2. *Slowly lift the leg above parallel and then lower it to tap your ankle to the roller without pausing. Slowly lift and lower 4 times while multitasking.*

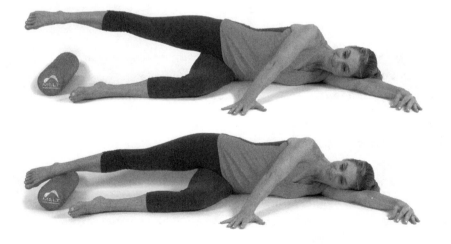

REPATTERN SET 2

1. *With the leg elevated, recheck your pelvic position (Tilt, Stack, and Roll) and rotate the leg in and out slowly and smoothly without pausing as you did in Reintegrate. Keep your pelvis and torso stable and still. Make sure you rotate the whole leg and not just the lower leg or foot.*

2. *Repeat 4 times while multitasking.*

You want to feel

+ *Fatigue or work in the upper region of the hip*

+ *Your leg wavering involuntarily*

Stop immediately if you feel

– *Fatigue or work in the calf, back strain, or low back pain*

– *Burning on the side of your thigh (the iliotibial [IT] band)*

– *Fatigue in the front of the hip joint rather than the outer hip region*

MELT Prep Sequence Helpers

▶ *Do any of these sequences first to prepare your body for Side Leg Lift: Seated Compression Sequence (page 170), Lower Body Rehydrate and Low Back Release Sequence (page 159), or Performance Foot Treatment (page 136).*

▶ *If you can't do Side Leg Lift, try Mini Bridge (page 229), Clams (page 216), or Inner Thigh Lift (page 220).*

Common Compensations

When the abductors are not firing properly, the common compensation is to move your pelvis and engage your external obliques and quadratus lumborum, above the waistline. To identify whether these muscles are overly involved, place your hand on your waistline to feel whether they engage when you move or lift the leg.

It's also common for the top leg to drift forward. The hip flexors will flex to compensate with other muscles. Instead, extend your leg slightly behind your torso but be mindful not to move your ribs forward.

Mini Bridge

The gluteus maximus is the largest muscle in your body. Eighty percent of this muscle attaches to the tensor fascia lata and your iliotibial band (important fascial tissues), and it helps with knee extension despite the muscle itself being way up in your hip. The other twenty percent, the deeper fibers, form an aponeurosis (dense fibrous connective tissue), which attaches directly to the gluteal tuberosity of the femur. These fibers help to stabilize and sustain force closure of the SI joint and supports its position during hip extension—essential to any athletic performance. These muscles are crucial in hip extension, rotation, abduction, and even adduction; sitting for long periods of time and daily repetitive postures, however, decrease their tone and supportive qualities.

Although the glutes are powerful muscles movers, their deepest aspects and "lower fibers" stabilize the pelvis in many ways—for example, when you're walking up stairs. To improve the supportive qualities and stability of your SI joint, Mini Bridge taps into the absolute end range of hip extension, often lost due to weakness in the deepest aspects of this tissue.

This is a great technique for people who have low back or neck pain, have had a C-section, postpartum pain, SI dysfunction, pelvic or hip pain, incontinence, and/or groin strain.

SETUP

1. *Lie on your back and put the roller under your pelvis, placing your feet hip-width apart.*

2. *Let your pelvis be neutral (try to avoid actively tucking it by practicing your modified tuck and tilt before you reintegrate) and keep your mid-ribs weighted to the floor. You can even interlace your fingers over your lower ribs to keep your ribs still.*

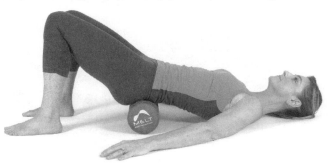

3. *Gently push your feet into the floor and find your core using your 3-D Breath. Think of the ball of your big toe, your outer foot, and your heel all compressed into the floor to activate the lower gluteal muscles, which are often inhibited to react to movement. Place your hands where your thighs meet your buttocks (the gluteal fold). If you have set up your position properly, you should feel the subtle engagement under your hands in your lower buttocks. Try not to "squeeze" your buttocks voluntarily. Just notice whether you can sense the subtle engagement.*

REINTEGRATE SET 1

1. *Push your feet into the floor to decompress your hips off the roller slightly and pause. Don't try to "lift" your pelvis from the roller; rather, decompress the weight of your hips from the roller. Remember, range isn't important. The objective is to get the lower fibers of your glutes to engage at the onset of the movement. Keep your hands around your gluteal fold to feel where the initiation should come from when you decompress the weight of your hips from the roller.*

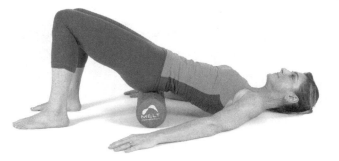

   – *Note incorrect posture (below) with back arched and a significantly higher lift of the pelvis.*

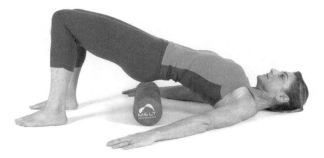

2. Next, think about sliding your heels away from the roller (no movement should occur, but this thought should bring slightly more weight to your ribs on the floor).

3. Then think about narrowing your knee angle by bringing your knees closer together by an inch.

4. Finally, think about energizing your knees over your toes, to lose the crease at the front of your hip joint entirely causing full hip extension.

5. Hold for 4 counts and slowly lower your pelvis and fully rest on the roller.

6. Repeat this sequence 4 times while multitasking with these ideas:

   – As you raise your hips, your feet get heavy and your pelvis gets light.

   – As you lower your hips, your feet get light and your pelvis gets heavy.

MULTITASK: *Your ribs and upper back are heavy and stable. Focus on your footing, keeping strong connection to both the outer region of your foot and your big toe mound. Place your hands on your ribs to focus on what's staying still as you move through end range hip extension.*

REPATTERN SET 1

1. Without releasing the contraction, lift and lower your pelvis, without arching your lower back, 4 times smoothly and slowly while multitasking.

2. Hold at the top where your hips are slightly lifted from the roller for 5 seconds before releasing fully.

ADD-ON CHALLENGE

1. Lift one leg to parallel, flex at the hip joint and knee bent, heel slack to the butt cheek as shown.

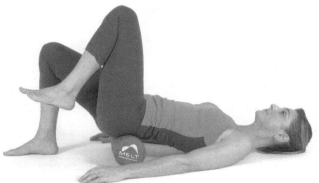

2. *Try to decompress the weight of your pelvis off the roller without shifting or laterally tilting your pelvis to either side.*

   – *Focus on lifting both sides of your pelvis equally.*

3. *Lift and lower your pelvis 4 times slowly and smoothly while multitasking. Rest for a moment.*

4. *Repeat on the other side.*

If you can't keep your pelvis level or your ribs heavy with only one foot on the floor, return to a double leg Mini Bridge.

You want to feel

+ *Fatigue or work in the lower buttocks (gluteal fold) and inner thigh*

Stop immediately if you feel

− *Pain or strain in the knees or low back*

− *Fatigue on the front of your thighs or cramping in the back of your thighs (hamstrings)*

MELT Prep Sequence Helpers

▶ *Do any of these sequences first to prepare your body for Mini Bridge: Lower Body Rehydrate and Low Back Release Sequence (page 159), Seated Compression Sequence (page 170), or Performance Foot Treatment (page 136).*

▶ *If you can't do Mini Bridge, try Core Challenge (page 233), Clams (page 216), or Side Leg Lift (page 229).*

Common Compensations

Arching the back and lifting the ribs to move the pelvis, and pressing the back of your arms into the floor to lift the hips. If the deep fibers of your glutes aren't in good timing, you will often get a hamstring cramp, the lower back extensors initiate the move, and/or low back ache or arching occurs during the motion. You may also find you feel pain in your knee, or your front thigh muscles burn and get fatigued. These are all signs of compensation.

◗ Core Challenge

Improving the control and timing of your NeuroCore can change your athleticism and reduce your risk of back and hip strain. This technique is *not* an "abdominal" exercise; rather, this move reintegrates the timing and co-coordination of the Reflexive Core and Rooted Core.

You are going to learn to sustain the Reflexive Core connection throughout the entire move. You'll also activate key spinal and pelvic stabilizers within the Rooted Core; one in particular—the psoas—needs to remain active throughout the move. However, its activation and contraction will change depending on where you are in the move.

The psoas will go through isometric (static contraction), eccentric (length contraction), and concentric (shortened contraction) engagement. As if you were "pumping" or massaging the tissues that connect the spine to the legs, this enhances the muscle's ability to keep your spine stable when you do any movements. When these stabilizing mechanisms of the NeuroCore are out of balance, you don't "not move"—rather, you compensate.

This technique can improve the control of these stabilizers and your overall stability. It's a challenging move. Use your breath and only move on the exhale when you first practice.

SETUP

1. *After doing the SI Joint Shear and Pelvic Tuck and Tilt Challenge, end with a subtle but active tilt position with your pelvis on the roller.*

2. *Bring your thighs nearly perpendicular to the floor, knees bent, lower legs slack to the butt cheeks.*

3. *Place your palms on your thighs so your fingertips are close to the knees. Elbows are straight.*

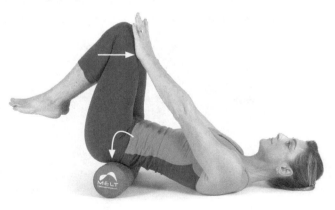

4. *Keep your pelvis in an active tilt on the top of the roller, ribs heavy and thighs pressing gently into your hands with your arms straight. Your ribs remain heavy between the shoulder blades, and the pelvis must remain in a tilt to sustain the natural curve of the low back. The weight of the tail triangle should remain on top of the roller.*

REINTEGRATE SET 1

1. *On an exhale, find your core using your* shhh, ssss, *or* haaa *sound. Keeping one thigh pressing into your palm, cross the opposite hand over so both hands are on the front of one thigh.*

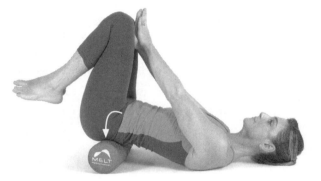

2. *Find your core and slowly move the opposite foot toward the floor with your knee remaining bent. Think of opening your hip and knee joint just enough to challenge the Rooted Core to activate properly. Sustain the rib and neutral pelvic position (slightly tilted on top of the roller) as you move the leg into a position where your foot is at the level of your roller, hovering over the floor. Pause for a moment as you take a shallow inhale without losing your core contact.*

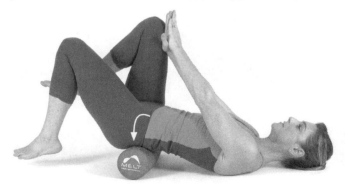

3. On an exhale, find your core again with your sound, press your thigh into your hand a little more without lifting your ribs or tucking the pelvis, and slowly return the lowered leg back to meet the hand without lifting your ribs or tucking the pelvis during the movement at all.

4. Place your hands on the other thigh and repeat the range of motion and control. Repeat 1 more time on both sides.

Note: *There is no Repattern with the Core Challenge.*

MULTITASK: *You must keep the position of the pelvis in a subtle tilt on the top of the roller. Do your best not to tuck your pelvis or flatten your low back at any point during this range. The bottom of the ribs stay heavy and differentiated from your pelvis in this range. Keep resistance of the thighs into your palm on one side. Focus on the action of your hip joint.*

Always precede this move with the SI Joint Shear and Pelvic Tuck and Tilt Challenge.

Once you get the hang of the move, try using a single exhale through the entire range rather than taking a breath between the down and up motion; repeat on the other side. Two times on both sides is plenty to reintegrate the NeuroCore. Don't overdo this move with more repetitions. You'll ultimately override the core reflex without knowing it and cause compensation.

You want to feel

+ *Connection in your torso and abdomen all the way to your spine*

Stop immediately if you feel

− *Burning in your hip joint or thigh, or pain in your low back. These are signs of compensation. If you feel fatigue in the front thigh of the posting leg, angle your thigh more toward your body to minimize compensation.*

MELT Prep Sequence Helpers

❯ *Do these moves first to prepare your body for the Core Challenge: SI Joint Shear (page 161) and Pelvic Tuck and Tilt Challenge (page 167).*

PART THREE

NeuroStrength Performance Sequences

N ow that you have the Four Rs of the MELT Protocol and Two Rs of Neuro-Strength under your belt and you've practiced the seven key NeuroStrength moves, we can put them together and create the fundamental sequences of MELT Performance—NeuroCore Stability, Upper Body Stability, and Lower Body Stability.

The beauty of these sequences is that they can benefit anyone, at any age, at any fitness level. Whether you're an elite athlete training for a specific sport, an athletic person looking to accelerate the healing process after an injury or surgery, someone who wants to reduce the risk of joint pain and add a proactive approach to self-care, or someone simply looking to reduce the negative side effects of a repetitive, daily lifestyle, these sequences are the ones to master. Once you become proficient at the sequences, you can try any of the MELT Maps presented in Part Four and know how to set yourself up and execute the moves with accuracy. You'll also know whether you're doing them right because you'll feel the fatigue in the specific areas of your body that each move is designed to reintegrate.

Even if you're an experienced, world-class athlete, the moves will still be very challenging at first because in a normal day, we don't consciously use the stabilizing mechanisms voluntarily. Furthermore, if we have compensatory pathways, it will take a few tries to reroute you back on the highway. Remember, it doesn't matter how muscularly strong you are; if you set yourself up properly and tune in to the reintegrative process, it should be challenging for *anyone* to do these NeuroStrength moves! If you find any of the moves to be easy or you don't feel them in a precise way, it's not because you're strong—it's most likely because your setup isn't correct.

Trust me, I know how an athlete's mind works because I spent many years of my life being an athlete and I've retrained many injured athletes and helped them restore their optimal performance. The desire to please others, gain praise, and feel strong are common to all athletes. You can't will or muscle your way through these techniques; if and when you do, as I've said already, you're simply cruising down a side street rather than getting on that neuro-highway. Remember, your inner athlete is waiting to reconnect with you. Give your utmost focus to that inner athlete and allow yourself to connect to your body in a whole new way.

▌ SEQUENCE BASICS

Accelerating Your Learning Curve

The three NeuroStrength sequences presented in Chapters 8, 9, and 10 will take you twenty to thirty minutes each when you first practice. The more familiar you are with the moves, the less time each sequence will take; it takes me ten to twenty minutes to do each of them. The NeuroCore Stability Sequence takes the least amount of time, followed by the Upper Body Stability Sequence and the Lower Body Stability Sequence. This timing is for the full sequences. In Part Four, you'll see how to select moves to create robust MELT Maps geared toward your specific needs and goals. For now, practice all the sequences and learn more about yourself.

How Often Should I Practice the Sequences?

Think of your month as three ten-day weeks. I want you to commit to practicing *each* of these sequences a minimum of once every ten days for the next sixty days. So basically, every third day, try one of the sequences. However, you can do one sequence every other day if you want to both accelerate your learning curve and refine your techniques. But don't do the same sequence more than every three days. Once you truly have NeuroStrength in your body, you can do the sequences less often yet sustain core, shoulder girdle, and pelvic girdle stability and control with less frequent intervention.

The All-Important Setup for the Sequences

If you need to review one of the moves with more specificity, go back to the chapter where it's presented step by step. For the Performance moves especially, the setup is essential, so if you need to go back and check out whether you've got it right, see the descriptions in Chapter 7.

Think of your sequences like flowing yoga poses. You'll go from one move to the next, and then to the next, flowing through each with focus and connection. Each of these sequences begins with a Rest Assess and ends with a Rest Reassess, letting you value the changes and allowing your Autopilot a moment to reset to an improved body baseline and reconnect to your center of gravity. It doesn't matter how great you get at doing the moves; you will always spend a moment scanning your body's current positioning to identify which common imbalances you notice before you jump into the next move. If you commit to memory the four most common imbalances on page 127, it shouldn't take you more than a couple of minutes to Rest Assess and Rest Reassess your body. Trust me, this is the secret sauce of restoring stability, so take the time to identify your current state and value the changes you can make for yourself.

After you've prepared the tissue with Rehydrate techniques, you'll do specific NeuroStrength moves that address the deep stabilizing mechanisms in that area of your body. Each of these moves will have three components, the Setup, Reintegrate Sets, and Repattern Sets. Remember these key concepts of each component.

Setup

- Make sure you have your pelvic or shoulder girdles in the right position. Focus on keeping your pelvis or shoulder girdle stable as you try to engage the stabilizing mechanisms. Draw your attention to what's staying stable rather than thinking about the movement you are going to create. Remember, NeuroStrength is not about strengthening muscles; it's about restoring neurological pathways of stability.

Reintegrate

- Reintegration involves a *small number of slow, precise movements*, pausing during and between each repetition. If you feel pain or strain while reintegrating, stop and start over. You've identified that you are having trouble reintegrating stability. Pain is your signal that you need to recheck your setup position, slow down, and practice Reintegration until you can do this part of the move with proper form and without pain.

- *You'll do only four Reintegrate repetitions.* If you feel you've found the stability pathway, move to the Repatterning set. If you sense pain or feel the activation of other regions of your body, stop and completely relax. Either wait for a moment and try to reset the position, or turn over and try the move on your other side. Interestingly, if one side of your body is inhibited, the other side may be more receptive. Go back to the side you had trouble with and try again, with even more focus on your setup and body position before you try executing the movement again.

Repattern

- Repatterning involves a small number of slow, precise movements, with *no pausing.* Repatterning restores the proper stability pathway, as well as control and motor timing, and reroutes your nervous system off the side streets and back onto the highway.

- The Repatterning sets have a *slightly faster pace, no pause, and greater difficulty* than the Reintegration sets, but it's still critical to stay focused on your setup position and what's staying stable during movement.

- Again, what's important to remember is it *takes only four repetitions* before the stabilizing mechanisms fatigue, causing compensation, so less is more. I guarantee, if you feel like you can do more reps, your nervous system is still using the shortcut, and in fact you're just strengthening the compensatory pathway.

When you put the moves together, you can achieve profound changes. I've seen and felt for myself and witnessed the effects of the sequences thousands of times. I want to send you off into trying these sequences with two basic goals: The short-term goal is to improve your Body Sense so you can more easily sense change; and the long-term goal is to improve your performance and resilience.

Finally, remember that your goal for using MELT is to enhance awareness as a foundation to improve your stability and the resilience of your performance. Don't become critical or judgmental when you sense imbalances or if you try a sequence and don't feel any change. Not noticing change also builds awareness! You'll soon learn that the order of moves in a sequence can entirely change the results.

Also, some sequences will create massive changes, and some, not so much. Perhaps one sequence doesn't seem to make any changes, but the next time you try it, you sense change—this is part of your mind-body reconnect! Truly, awareness is half the battle of proactive self-care. We wait until we really feel problems instead of identifying the common imbalances or pre-pain signals that you now know all about. Because you have this understanding through the Autopilot Assessments and Rest Assess, you've got all the tools you need to exceed your fitness goals.

Perfection is an unachievable goal, which can leave you feeling frustrated. But you are already amazing. I know this because I'm like you. If that weren't true, you wouldn't have gotten to this part of the book. You are a seeker of betterment and well-being. You are far beyond average. Ground yourself in that knowledge as you give your neurological stability mechanisms a boost.

I'll say it again: Practice isn't about perfection—it's about enhancing your body's natural ability to function with efficiency and resilience. Practice builds essential awareness. The more aware you are of your current state, and the more aware you are of where you want to go, the faster you can get there.

Becoming a hands-off bodyworker in and of itself is a skill to acquire. You may want to do these sequences in front of a mirror to refine your skills. Although using your vision to see compensation can help you acquire the right setup, our objective is to improve your Body Sense. So after you feel the work in the right places, take the time to focus inward, taking visual cues away to gain the full benefits of the method.

8

NeuroCore Stability Sequence

Most of us have some level of NeuroCore imbalance due to daily living. Can sitting at a desk with your pelvis tucked under inhibit the NeuroCore and ultimately cause low back pain? Does poor diet cause gut issues that lead to poor reflexive integrity? Can overtraining your abdominal muscles cause the mechanisms to become faulty? Yes! Regardless of how NeuroCore imbalance begins, it's happening to a lot of us.

The primary goal of this sequence is to rebalance and reintegrate the timing of the Reflexive Core and the Rooted Core mechanisms to improve spinal mobility, gut support, and pelvic stability and control. For best results, tune into your core activation and focus on what's staying stable the moment before and as you move.

Rest Assess

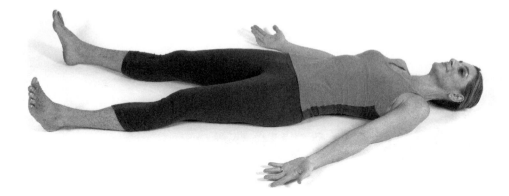

1. *Use your Body Sense to scan your masses and spaces for stuck stress, and notice any imbalances. Turn your head left to right to identify restrictions in your neck space; touch your navel if you need a reference point to identify an excessive arch in your lower back space.*

2. *Notice your left and right sides from ear to heel. Does your Autopilot have a clear connection to your center of gravity (your pelvis) before you get started? Do you feel balanced from left to right?*

3. *Notice and remember what you feel.*

SI Joint Shear

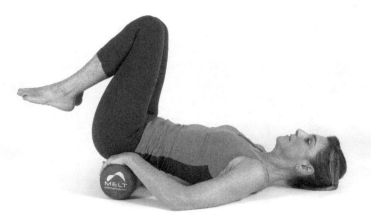

SETUP

1. *The center of your pelvis is on the top of the roller. Your knees are bent and slightly angled toward your torso.*

2. *Tip your knees slightly left to right 5 to 10 times.*

MOVE

1. *Keep your knees tipped to the left and begin to shear your left SI joint by creating small circles with both legs, or just your left leg, or march your knees forward and back 4 to 6 times each.*

2. *Pause on the left SI joint and take two focused breaths. Repeat on the right side.*

3. *Bring your knees back to the center.*

Bent Knee Press

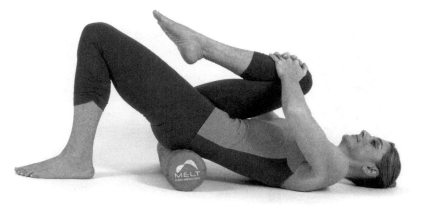

SETUP

1. *The center of your pelvis is on the top of the roller. Place your left foot on the floor, knee bent.*

2. *Keep your focus on actively tucking your pelvis.*

3. *Bring your right knee toward your chest. Interlace your fingers either around your right shin or under your right thigh.*

4. *Keep your left thigh aligned with your hip and your knee pointed straight ahead like a headlight. Keep your hips square.*

MOVE

1. *Take a focused breath, and on the exhale, further accentuate the tuck of your pelvis by using your hands to draw your right knee toward your nose while your left knee gets energized toward your left toes.*

2. *Inhale, ease back your lengthening intention, and on the exhale increase the tensional pull again.*

3. *Release your right leg and set your right foot on the floor. Repeat on the other side.*

Hip to Heel Press

SETUP

1. *The center of your pelvis is on the top of the roller. Place your left foot on the floor, knee bent.*

2. *Your pelvis is in a tilt; your knee must remain fully extended.*

3. *Extend your right leg to parallel, flex your ankle, and keep your left foot light on the floor.*

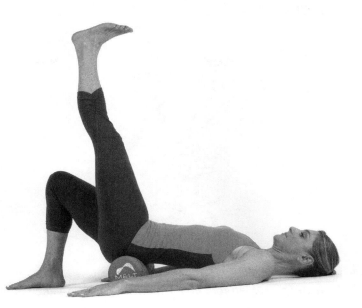

MOVE

1. *Without bending your knee, flex at your hip to move your right leg toward perpendicular to the roller but stop just prior to perpendicular or where your knee wants to bend.*

2. *On your exhale increase the tensional pull by flexing your ankle and accentuating your tilt onto the top of the roller. Inhale and ease back the intentional length and repeat again.*

3. *Release your right leg and set your right foot on the floor. Repeat on the other side.*

Figure 4

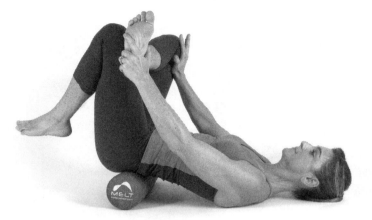

1. *Keep your left foot on the floor with your left knee bent. Flex your right ankle and cross it over the left thigh; find your core as you bring your legs into your chest.*

2. *Keep your hips stable and ensure you don't laterally side bend at your waistline. Use your left hand either on your right foot or behind the left thigh to sustain proper positioning. Create the "push-press" in equal tension: Use your right hand to push your right thigh away from the hip socket, and with equal pressure press your left thigh into your right ankle.*

3. *Once you achieve this "push-press" position, tilt your pelvis on top of the roller to open the hip joint and find length. Inhale and ease back the tensional length; on the exhale, try again to tilt your pelvis on top of the roller without excessively arching your back as you push your right knee away from your hip joint and press your left knee toward your right ankle with equal effort.*

4. *Set your left foot back to the floor, release your right leg, and repeat on the other side.*

Pelvic Tuck and Tilt Challenge

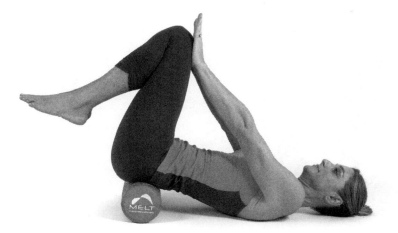

SETUP

1. *The roller is still under your pelvis. Bring your thighs toward your chest, knees bent. Place your hands on your thighs and push them away from your chest until your arms are straight.*

2. *Gently compress your thighs toward your hands and allow your mid-rib wall, just below your shoulder girdle, to sink toward the floor.*

MOVE

1. *Sustain both points of active compression, thighs to hands, ribs to the floor. On an exhale, focus on differentiating your pelvis from your ribs and hip joint by tucking your pelvis without letting your arms bend, then tilting your pelvis back to the top of the roller without decreasing your thigh-to-hand pressure or moving your ribs off the floor.*

2. *Take another inhale, and on each exhale move through your Tuck and Tilt 4 to 6 times.*

Core Challenge

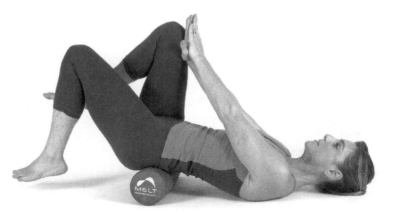

SETUP

1. *The roller is still under your pelvis at its center. Gently press your right thigh into your hand, keep your ribs heavy and still on the floor, and tilt your pelvis to the top of the roller. Heels stay slack to your buttocks.*

REINTEGRATE

1. On an exhale, allow your left hip joint to open, slowly lowering your left foot toward the floor with your knee remaining bent.

2. *Pause in that position, ensuring that your setup has remained the same, and on an exhale, slowly return your left leg to the original position. Repeat on both sides two times.*

You want to feel

+ *Connection in your torso and abdomen all the way to your spine*

Stop immediately if you feel

− *Burning in your hip joint or thigh, or pain in your low back. These are signs of compensation. If you feel fatigue in the front thigh of the posting leg, angle your thigh slightly more toward your body to minimize compensation.*

Mini Bridge

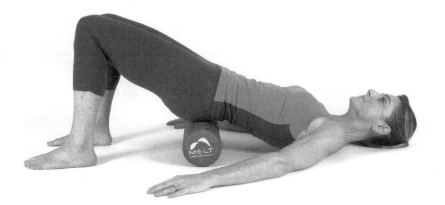

SETUP

1. *Place your feet hip-width apart, knees bent, pelvis relaxed in your neutral position. You can always use the Modified Tuck and Tilt Challenge to set up your position.*

2. *Focus on what's staying stable: Keep your mid-rib wall relaxed and heavy on the floor, below your shoulder blades, with your core engaged.*

REINTEGRATE

1. *Find solid footing; your feet get heavy and hips get light as you decompress the weight of your hips off the roller. Once you are in this position, multitask with minimal movement for 10 to 15 seconds:*

   – *Energize your heels away from your hips to bring more weight to your rib wall.*

   – *Narrow your knee angle by 1 inch.*

   – *Energize your knees over your toes.*

   – *Hold this end position for 5 seconds.*

2. *Fully release your pelvis on top of the roller (hips get heavy, feet get light), take a focused breath, find your core, and repeat 3 more times.*

REPATTERN

1. *Without releasing the contraction, lift and lower your pelvis 4 times while you multitask—energize heels away from hips, narrow knees, knees over toes as a constant state of focus, ribs heavy and stationary.*

   - **ADD-ON CHALLENGE:** *Bring one thigh to perpendicular to the roller, knee bent, and using only one leg, lift the weight of your hips off the roller, keeping your pelvis level. Lift and lower 4 times and repeat on the other side.*

You want to feel

  + *The work in your lower buttocks and inner thigh*

Stop immediately if you feel

  – *Fatigue in your front thigh, pain in your knees or low back, or cramping in the back of your thigh*

Rest Reassess

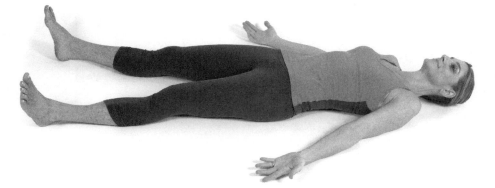

1. Use your *Body Sense* to scan your masses and spaces; notice whether you have decreased any imbalances.

   - Are your ribs, pelvis, and thighs more relaxed on the floor? Is your low back less tense and arched? Can you turn your head more efficiently?

2. Does your *Autopilot* have a clear connection to your center of gravity?

   - Do you feel more even from left to right?

3. Notice and remember what you feel.

9

Upper Body
Stability Sequence

Daily habitual activities like working at your computer, using your smartphone, carrying a backpack, or training for a sport cause many faulty patterns, as well as unwanted tension and stiffness in the upper body. Beyond that, our torso is often flexed and fixated, leading the cervical spine to become hypermobile and our shoulder girdle to lose its integrity. All of this is a common cause of aches and pains.

The primary goal of this sequence is to restore stability, control, and mobility of your shoulder girdle, cervical and thoracic spine, and shoulder joints. For best results, tune into your core activation and focus on what's staying stable the moment before and as you move.

Rest Assess

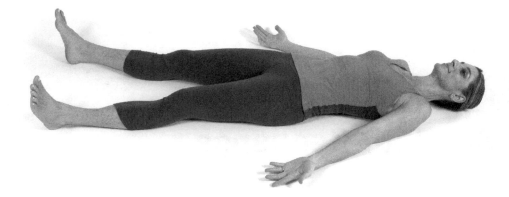

1. *Use your Body Sense to scan your masses and spaces for stuck stress, and notice any imbalances.*

2. *Does your Autopilot have a clear connection to your center of gravity (your pelvis) before you get started?*

3. *Notice and remember what you feel.*

Rib Length Assess

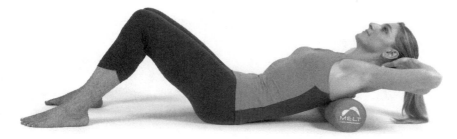

SETUP

1. *Rest your shoulder blades on the roller, knees bent, hands behind your head, elbows open and wide. Keep your pelvis in a tuck. Gently press your head in your hands to avoid extending your neck as you move.*

MOVE

1. *Curl your ribs forward into flexion to properly set up your lower ribs. Focus on your bottom ribs staying still as you move to extension. Avoid pulling your head forward or changing your neck position.*

2. *As you exhale, extend your ribs toward the top of the roller. Your low back and neck remain still—avoid hyperextending your spaces.*

3. *Notice any tension through your chest as you inhale. As you exhale, return to rib flexion. Repeat 2 times.*

4. *On your second repetition, remain in extension and assess your ability to side bend only your ribs left and right, pausing on either side for a focused breath to evaluate any tension or restrictions in your torso. Return to center, take a focused breath, and return to rib flexion.*

Upper Back Glide and Shear

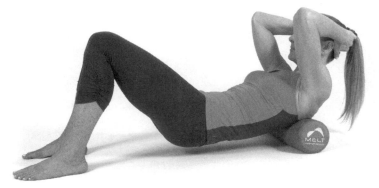

SETUP

1. *Rest your upper back on the roller, hands behind your head, neck relaxed, elbows pointed forward, ribs flexed, pelvis in a tuck.*

MOVE

1. *Engage your core, lift your hips slightly off the floor, and begin gliding your upper back between your shoulder blades in small controlled movements to identify any tender regions, or barriers.*

2. *Find a tolerable spot to compress, stop moving, set your tucked pelvis back to the floor, and curl your torso slightly more into flexion to Shear. Compress and twist by tipping your torso slightly left and right 4 to 5 times, as if opening a child-proof bottle cap. Keep the movement small.*

3. *Wait to allow the tissue a moment to adapt, then lift your hips, move the roller lower toward the bottom of your shoulder blades, in the mid rib region or bra line by pushing into your feet, find a new spot, and repeat the Glide and Shear again.*

Note: *You can perform the next four Glide and Shear moves all on one side, then return to center and repeat all four on the other side. You can do some or all four moves back to back or skip some or all of the compression moves and go directly to Upper Back Rinse, depending on your time and ability. Add more moves as you become more comfortable moving your body on the roller.*

Inner Shoulder Blade Glide and Shear

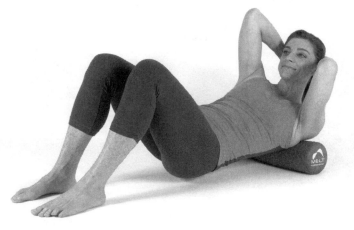

SETUP

1. *Rest your upper back on the roller, hands behind your head, neck relaxed, elbows pointed forward, ribs flexed, pelvis in a tuck.*

2. *Keep your core engaged, tip your upper body slightly to the left, and lift your hips slightly off the floor.*

MOVE

1. *Glide the tip and inside edge of your left shoulder blade, using your feet to move your body forward and back. Meet the barrier, stop moving, set your left buttock back to the floor, and begin your Shear.*

2. *Reach your arm up and out anywhere in front of you to stimulate the tissue between your shoulder blade and shoulder joint 4 to 5 times.*

3. *Remember, if you have neck pain, move your arm in and out 4 to 5 times with your hand on your head. If you have shoulder pain, place your hand on your shoulder and move your arm in front of your body with your elbow bent 4 to 5 times to modify the Shear.*

4. *With your head resting in your hand, pause and give the tissue a moment to adapt. Repeat on the other side or add the next move.*

Side Rib Glide and Outer Shoulder Blade Glide and Shear

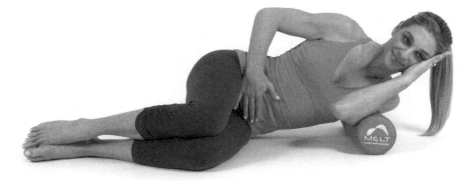

SETUP

1. *Lie on your left side with the bottom of your shoulder blade and mid-rib wall resting on the roller. Rest your forearm and side of your left arm on the roller, and rest your head in your right hand to relax your neck.*

MOVE

1. *Glide your side ribs by curling your torso into flexion and returning to extension 5 to 10 times, then pause on a spot where you can tolerate the pressure and take two focused breaths, finding your core on each exhale.*

2. *Glide your outer shoulder blade by tipping your torso back slightly so your left elbow angles more toward the ceiling and the roller compresses the bottom and outer edge of your shoulder blade. Gently side bend your torso to move the roller up and down the outer edge of your shoulder blade 5 to 10 times, exploring the area for barriers or tenderness.*

3. *Open and close your bottom arm toward and away from your face with your hand supporting your head, or release your hand and arc your arm over the roller to both sides like a rainbow 4 to 5 times.*

4. *Return your hand to your head, relax, take two focused breaths, and allow the tissue time to adapt. Repeat on other side or continue to Arm Glide and Shear.*

Arm Glide and Shear

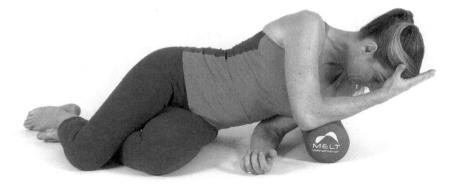

SETUP

1. Rest your left upper arm on the roller at the bottom of your deltoid. Rest your head on your right hand to reduce strain in the neck.

MOVE

1. Glide the side of your arm by flexing and extending your torso in and away from your belly to investigate the tissue for barriers.

2. Meet a barrier, edge up against it, and prepare to Shear.

3. Indirect Shear: Lift and lower your forearm off the floor by rotating at the shoulder joint so your arm moves toward your belly and return 4 to 5 times.

4. Direct Shear: Keep your forearm on the floor and punch your arm forward and back 4 to 5 times.

5. Relax, take two focused breaths, and allow the tissue a moment to adapt. Repeat on other side or continue to Chest Glide and Shear.

Chest Glide and Shear

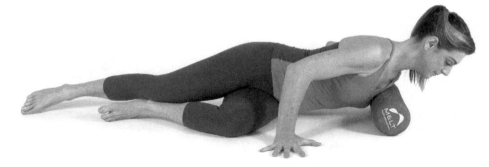

SETUP

1. *Place the front of your left shoulder and chest on the roller; your left arm is behind you, palm down. Place your head in your right hand if you feel tension in your neck, or keep both hands on the floor, palms down.*

MOVE

1. *Use one or both hands on the floor and your core to help you move the roller up toward the bottom of your collar bone; your body curls in slightly. Then extend your torso forward; the roller moves downward. Repeat this motion 5 to 10 times and investigate for barriers. Find a tolerable spot, edging just against the barrier, and Shear.*

2. *Shear your chest by shifting your torso slightly left to right 4 to 5 times. Remember, you aren't rubbing your skin against the roller; you're pinning the flesh against the roller and Shearing the underside against your ribs.*

3. *Pause and take two focused breaths, allowing your body to sink into the roller and giving the tissue time to adapt on each exhale.*

Either repeat on the other side or, if you've done all the moves on one side, return to your beginning position, with your mid-back on the roller, and repeat the above four Glide and Shear moves on the other side.

Upper Back Rinse

SETUP

1. *Rest your mid-back on the roller, hands behind your head for support, elbow angled inward, torso slightly flexed.*

2. *Find your core, set your feet slightly in front of your knees, lift your hips an inch off the floor, and bring your knees atop your ankles to set up the roller to your upper back.*

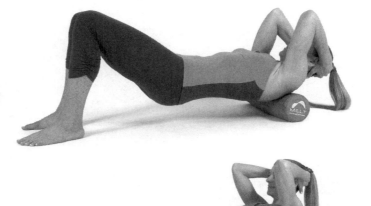

MOVE

1. *Take a focused breath. On the exhale, engage your core, keep your hips low, push into your feet to allow the roller to slowly travel down your torso with your ribs flexed. Keep consistent pressure as your legs extend and your hips settle back to the floor; the roller moves down your back, just below your bra line or shoulder blades.*

2. *Reset your feet slightly in front of your knees and then find your core, lift your hips off the floor, and bring your knees over your feet again so the roller moves to your upper back. Pause and take a focused breath.*

3. *Repeat the Rinse 3 to 4 times to improve fluid flow throughout your body.*

Note: *You can do either or both Side Lying Arm Fans and Side Lying Backhand on one side, then flip over and repeat on the other side. The resistance band is under your hips for both moves.*

Side Lying Arm Fans

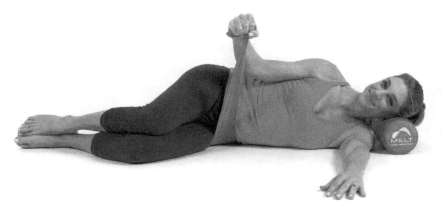

SETUP

1. *Lie comfortably on your left side with the resistance band under your left hip. Bend your knees and hips at approximately 45 degrees. Reach the left arm out slightly so you're lying on the outer shoulder blade, not your shoulder joint. You should be lying on your outer thigh more than the side of your hip bone.*

2. *Place your right elbow on your right hip and internally rotate your arm at your shoulder joint until you find your fingertips on the band.*

3. *Crumple up the band to make a handle, and pull up on the band with your forearm parallel to the floor and wrist in line with your forearm.*

REINTEGRATE SET 1

1. *Punch your arm forward and back 4 times to set up your angle, ensuring that your hand remains in front of your hip throughout the range of motion.*

2. *Return your arm back toward your hip, but stop before you touch your hip with your elbow. Hold this position for 10 to 15 seconds and allow the reintegration to take effect.*

REINTEGRATE SET 2

1. *Externally rotate your arm from your shoulder joint, keeping your wrist in line with your forearm, pausing at the top for 2 counts. Then slowly lower to the parallel starting position, and again, pause for 2 counts. Repeat this 4 times.*

REPATTERN

1. *Externally rotate your arm 4 times at a consistent pace, with no pausing. Then let go of the band and repeat, slightly increasing the range of motion, 4 times.*

You want to feel

+ *Fatigue or burning in the shoulder joint and rear upper arm*

Stop immediately if you feel

− *Strain or pain in the neck, collarbone, forearms, biceps, or wrist*

Repeat this on the other side or continue to Side Lying Backhand.

Side Lying Backhand

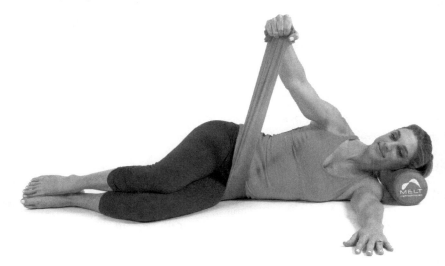

SETUP

1. *Lie on your side comfortably with the resistance band under your left hip. Raise up your right arm and move your shoulder girdle down the side of your ribs so your neck space feels open and relaxed. Angle your arm slightly toward your hip.*

2. *Keep your ribs still and reach your straight arm down to the floor to find the band. Crumple up the band like a handle and pull it up, bringing your arm parallel to the floor, hand angled slightly toward your hips rather than out in front of your shoulder joint.*

REINTEGRATE SET 1

1. *Move your arm forward and back 4 times slowly so your forearm travels over your hips when your elbow bends, as you did in Side Lying Arm Fans; then as the elbow straightens, punch your arm forward and out, hand staying in front of the hips. On your final repetition, hold your arm straight, hand angled in front of your hips. Hold this position for 10 to 15 seconds.*

REINTEGRATE SET 2

1. *With your arm straight and hand angled in front of your hips, slowly increase tension on the band by pulling upward, like lifting a bucket of water, away from the floor. Pause for 2 counts, and then slowly lower to the parallel starting position; pause for 2 counts. Repeat this 4 times.*

REPATTERN

1. *In the same range of motion, slightly increase the pace without pausing at either end range; repeat 4 times. Then release the band and repeat 4 times, slightly increasing the range of motion.*

You want to feel

+ *Fatigue or burning in the back and front of the shoulder joint and rear upper arm*

Stop immediately if you feel

− *Strain or pain in the neck, collarbones, forearms, biceps, or wrist*

Repeat on the other side.

Rib Length Reassess

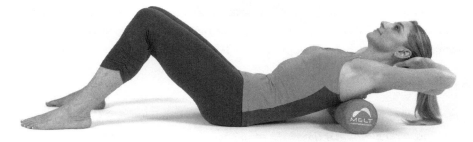

1. *Return your mid-ribs to the roller and reassess your ability to differentiate your ribs from your neck and low back. Tuck your pelvis and curl your ribs into flexion, then extend your ribs to the top of the roller.*

2. *Take two focused breaths and notice whether your range has increased and you feel less restriction in your torso.*

3. *Find your core on each exhale to enhance the lengthening.*

4. *Repeat flexion to extension 2 times, pausing at the extended position for two breaths.*

5. *Stay in extension and side bend left and right, noticing whether you've increased range or decreased restriction. Pause on both sides and take two focused breaths to enhance the length and mobility of your torso.*

6. *Return to the center, move the roller away, and do a Rest Reassess.*

Rest Reassess

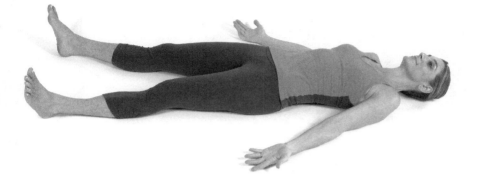

1. *Scan your masses and spaces and notice whether you decreased any imbalances.*

   – *Are your ribs, pelvis, and thighs more relaxed on the floor? Is your low back less tense and arched? Can you turn your head more efficiently?*

2. *Does your Autopilot have a clear connection to your center of gravity?*

   – *Do you feel more even from left to right?*

3. *Notice and remember what you feel.*

10

Lower Body Stability Sequence

The stabilizing mechanisms of the lower body are often inhibited by overuse and misuse of the superficial movers, which are trained for strength and power.

The primary goal of this sequence is to restore stability and control to the pelvic girdle. Frequently check in and reset your pelvic position to reduce compensation and faulty patterning. For best results, tune into your core activation and focus on what's staying stable the moment before and as you move.

Rest Assess

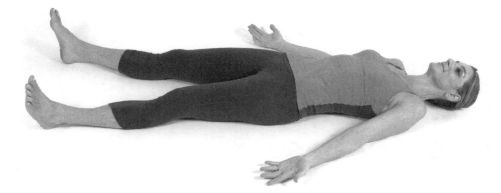

1. *Scan your masses and spaces for stuck stress and notice any imbalances.*

2. *Does your Autopilot have a clear connection to your center of gravity (your pelvis) before you get started?*

3. *Notice and remember what you feel.*

Deep Hip Glide and Shear

SETUP

1. *Sit on top of the roller, knees bent, feet flat on the floor. Place your fingers on the floor in front of the roller for balance.*

2. *Using your feet, move your pelvis over the roller, so the roller moves forward and back over the bottom of your pelvis and sits bones 5 to 10 times.*

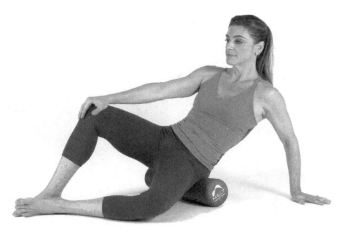

MOVE

1. *Tip your body toward the left side and place your left hand on the floor behind the roller for balance; rest your right hand on your knees. Using your feet, Glide by moving the roller forward and back along the outer edge of your left sits bone where your deep hip muscles reside, 5 to 10 times. Explore the deep hip for barriers.*

   - *To increase the compression on your deep hip, open your left hip joint into external rotation, allow the deep hip muscles to sink more deeply into the roller, and continue to Glide, pressing mostly into your right foot.*

2. *Meet a barrier by edging up against it and Shearing.*

   - **INDIRECT SHEAR:** *Moving at the hip joint, clam the leg up and down 4 to 5 times, then pause and take a focused breath or try a Direct Shear.*

   - **DIRECT SHEAR:** *Straighten your left leg and roll your hip forward and back over the roller 4 to 5 times. Pause with a focused breath and allow the tissue a moment to adapt.*

3. *Repeat on the other side.*

Tail Triangle and SI Joint Glide

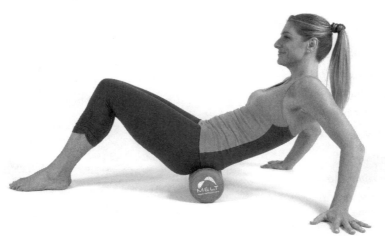

SETUP

1. *Place both hands on the floor behind the roller, hands wide, fingers pointed outward. Keep your ribs relaxed and heavy, pelvis in a tuck, knees bent. Think about keeping your hands and feet light on the floor to engage your core.*

MOVE

1. *Glide your tail triangle (sacrum) by moving your body forward and back so the roller moves up and down the back of your pelvis 5 to 10 times. Keep your core engaged as you move.*

2. *Glide your left SI joint by tipping your knees slightly to the left (think of the face of a clock and tip your knees to 11 o'clock only). Use your feet to move the roller up and down your left SI joint 5 to 10 times.*

3. *Glide your right SI joint by tipping your knees slightly right, and repeat the gliding motion 5 to 10 times. Then return to the center.*

Side Hip Glide and Shear

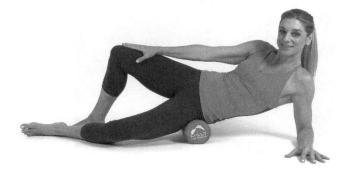

SETUP

1. *Place your left forearm on the floor behind the roller, knees bent, allowing the roller to compress the side of your left hip; place your right hand on your thighs or knees to help you control the movement of the Glide.*

MOVE

1. *Using your feet, move the roller up and down the side of your hip 5 to 10 times and explore the region for barriers.*

   – *To increase pressure, you can drop your left thigh down to the floor and use mostly your right foot to navigate the Gliding motion up and down the left hip. The more relaxed you are, the more you will affect the tissue all the way to your hip bone.*

2. *Meet your barrier, edge up against it, and Shear.*

   – **INDIRECT SHEAR:** *With your left foot on the floor, create internal and external rotation at the hip joint, clamming the leg in and out 4 to 5 times.*

   – **DIRECT SHEAR:** *Straighten your left knee and allow your entire body to roll forward and back over the roller. If you feel like you are going over a speed bump or losing pressure against the barrier, lean slightly forward and create cross-friction by shifting your hips forward and back 4 to 5 times. Remember, you aren't rubbing your skin on the roller; you're twisting the flesh against the bone by pinning your skin atop the roller as you move.*

3. *Pause, take a focused breath, and allow the tissue a moment to adapt.*

4. *Repeat on your other side.*

Clams

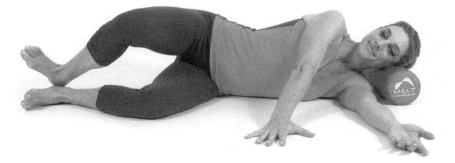

SETUP

1. *Lie comfortably on your side, bottom arm reached out slightly so you're lying on your ribs rather than your arm. Shift your bottom hip back slightly so you feel more weight resting on the outer thigh rather than the hip.*

2. *Find your Tilt, Stack, and Roll, and engage your core.*

REINTEGRATE SET 1

1. *Keep your heels together and clam your top leg without rolling your top hip back. You can keep your top hand on your hip and use touch to focus on keeping your hip still as you move your top leg upward.*

2. *Pause in the clam position and reset your Tilt, Stack, and Roll. Hold this position for 10 seconds.*

3. *Sustain the pose, place your top hand on the floor, and try to decompress the weight of your bottom thigh from the floor. Hold this pose for another 10 seconds, then rest the lower leg back to the floor. Recheck your Tilt, Stack, and Roll and take a focused breath.*

REINTEGRATE SET 2

1. *Slowly lower your top thigh to your bottom thigh, but don't relax. Clam the top thigh again, heels together, pelvis in the Tilt, Stack, and Roll position; pause at the top for 4 counts and then slowly return. Repeat 4 times, pausing at the end range each time.*

REPATTERN

1. *Repeat the motion 4 times smoothly without the pause.*

2. *Repeat on the other side.*

You want to feel

+ *Fatigue in the lower hip region*

Stop immediately if you feel

− *Fatigue in the front thigh, low back, or neck*

Inner Thigh Lift

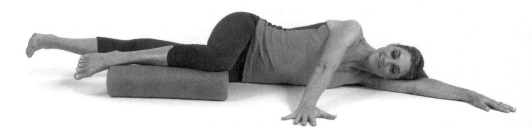

SETUP

1. *Lying on one side, place the shin of your top leg on top of the roller, knee bent, bottom leg straight. Find a slight tilt, keeping the ribs stable. Stack your top hip slightly. Take a focused breath and find your core.*

REINTEGRATE SET 1

1. *Reach your bottom leg long and slowly lift it from the floor while keeping your pelvis stable; then angle the bottom leg toward the roller a few inches so your bottom hip joint is slightly flexed.*

2. *Check for compensation by placing your top hand on the floor; then subtly lighten the weight of your top calf from the roller and lift your bottom leg up 1 inch more. Hold this for 4 seconds, then rest your top calf back on the roller and sustain the pose for a total of 30 seconds.*

REINTEGRATE SET 2

1. *With your bottom leg still lifted, try to lift a few inches higher, pause for 2 counts, and lower your leg halfway to the floor. Pause and repeat the range 4 times, pausing at both ends of the movement.*

REPATTERN SET 1

1. *Slowly lower your leg all the way to the floor and lift to your top range 4 times with no pause.*

REPATTERN SET 2

1. *At the top range, lift and lower the leg 1 inch in a slow, controlled pulsing motion, 4 times. Hold at the top range for 2 counts before releasing your leg to the floor.*

You want to feel

+ *Fatigue or work in the inner thigh, closer to the hip*

Stop immediately if you feel

− *Pain or strain in the knee or low back*

− *Engagement in the muscles above the pelvis at the waistline*

Remain on this side and try Side Leg Lift before turning over to repeat both moves.

Side Leg Lift

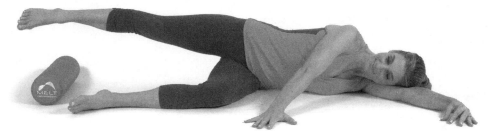

SETUP

1. *Lie comfortably on your side, bottom arm reached out so you aren't lying on your shoulder. Bend the bottom knee at 90 degrees. You want to feel that you're lying on your outer thigh rather than on your hip bone. Place the roller under your top leg near your ankle.*

2. *Find your Tilt, Stack, and Roll with your top hand on your hip, and find your core.*

REINTEGRATE SET 1

1. *Keep your pelvis stable and slowly lift your top leg so that it's parallel to the floor, with your leg in line with your torso. Avoid flexing the hip joint. Reset your Tilt, Stack, and Roll and hold this position for 10 to 15 seconds.*

2. *Now internally rotate your leg and pause for 2 counts; then externally rotate your leg from your hip joint, keeping your pelvis stable, and pause for 2 counts. Repeat this rotation 4 times, focusing on keeping your pelvis still and in the Tilt, Stack, and Roll position.*

REINTEGRATE SET 2

1. *Recheck your pelvic position, keep your thigh slightly internally rotated, and then lift your leg 1 inch higher and pause for 2 counts. Lower your thigh just to parallel, and pause for 2 counts. Repeat this small range of motion 4 times.*

REPATTERN SET 1

1. *Recheck your Tilt, Stack, and Roll. Slowly lift the leg above parallel and then lower it down until your ankle hits the roller; slowly lift again through the full range, with no pause, 4 times.*

REPATTERN SET 2

1. *Lift your leg to your end range, about 1 inch higher than parallel, with your pelvis remaining in the optimal position; create internal-to-external rotation 4 times with no pause.*

You want to feel

+ *Fatigue or work in the upper region of the hip*

+ *Your leg wavering involuntarily*

Stop immediately if you feel

− *Fatigue or work in the calf, back strain, or low back pain*

− *Burning on the side of your thigh (the iliotibial [IT] band)*

− *Fatigue in the front of the hip joint rather than the outer hip region*

Turn over and try the Inner Thigh Lift and Side Leg Lift on the other side.

Rest Reassess

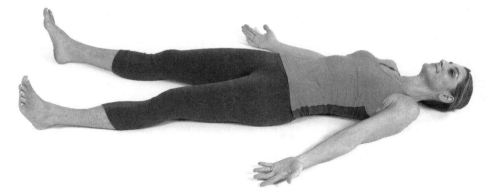

1. *Scan your masses and spaces and notice whether you decreased any imbalances.*

   – *Are your ribs, pelvis, and thighs more relaxed on the floor? Is your low back less tense and arched? Can you turn your head more efficiently?*

2. *Does your Autopilot have a clear connection to your center of gravity?*

   – *Do you feel more even from left to right?*

3. *Notice and remember what you feel.*

PART FOUR

NeuroStrength Performance Maps

11

Stability Maps

Now that you've tried the fundamental sequences of MELT Performance, you can put the moves together to devise new MELT Maps. To get you started, I've created some basic Maps so you can see how to mix and match moves to help you improve your stability and performance and reach higher goals.

I've broken down the Maps into three categories: Sports Performance Maps, Pain and Joint Injury Maps, and Lifestyle Maps. You can try any of these Maps, even if you don't play basketball, for example, or you have had a recent hip replacement, or you have a desk job. Also remember that the moves in this book are the most important NeuroStrength moves to master—but they aren't *all* the moves. There's plenty more to learn! Once you've tried these sequences, you can watch them on MELT On Demand. There, you'll find streaming video tutorials, sequences, and Maps in these categories to help you learn more and refine your techniques.

Many sports have both Training Day and Game/Performance Day Maps. The difference is important: On game days, you want to focus on rehydration moves to improve agility and grounding, whereas on training days, you want to focus on joint stability and NeuroStrength moves. Knowing when to do which types of sequences is the secret to enhancing sports performance.

I've included more than a dozen different Maps in this chapter. Each is similar, but the moves are ordered differently for a specific reason. Start with the category you think most specifically represents your lifestyle and goals, and then try some of the other Maps. I also suggest that you keep a journal to track your results.

▶ Sports Performance Maps

Although every sport has its own specifics, many require similar stability. For example, whether your sport is baseball, golf, tennis, or Frisbee, you know that grip strength, rotational control, and ground reaction force are essential.

I've worked with thousands of athletes, amateurs and professionals. Even though dancing, volleyball, and basketball have different muscular strength needs, the lateral stability required to jump and land with good timing and the shoulder stability necessary for movement accuracy are very similar. Common injuries are ankle and lateral knee sprains, not to mention chronic low back and neck pain. To avoid these common mishaps and improve lateral agility and stability, similar Performance Maps can be created.

Start by using the Maps that best represent your sport, then try the others and track your results. Remember, regardless of their sport, all athletes need grip strength and accurate ground reaction force timing, as well as a stable yet mobile neck. The MELT Performance Hand and Foot Treatments should be your go-to treatments on training days, and the MELT Mini Performance Hand and Foot Treatments are great for game days no matter the sport you love to play. I personally do the Neck Release Sequence before bedtime each night to get a more restful night's sleep and to keep my neck pain-free.

Maps for Basketball, Dance, Gymnastics, Skating, Volleyball, and Mixed Martial Arts

Training Day Map (approximately 30 minutes)

Rest Assess

Performance Hand Treatment

Seated Compression Sequence

Side Leg Lift

Side Lying Arm Fans

Inner Thigh Lift

Repeat Side Leg Lift, Side Lying Arm Fans, and Inner Thigh Lift on the other side.

Rest Reassess

SI Joint Shear

Bent Knee Press

Mini Bridge

Pelvic Tuck and Tilt Challenge

Core Challenge

Rest Reassess

Game Day Map (approximately 12 minutes)

Rest Assess

> *If you have an extra 5 minutes, do a Mini Performance Foot Treatment after the Rest Assess.*

Deep Hip Glide and Shear

SI Joint Shear

Pelvic Tuck and Tilt Challenge

Core Challenge

Figure 4

Rest Reassess

Maps for Football, Soccer/Rugby, Ice Hockey, and Skiing/Snowboarding

Training Day Map (approximately 25 minutes)

Rest Assess

Performance Foot Treatment

Tail Triangle and SI Joint Glide

Deep Hip Glide and Shear

Clams

Inner Thigh Lift

Rest Reassess

SI Joint Shear

Pelvic Tuck and Tilt Challenge

Core Challenge

Bent Knee Press

Rest Reassess

Game Day Map (approximately 12 minutes)

Rest Assess

If you have an extra 5 minutes, add a Mini Performance Hand Treatment after the Rest Assess.

Tail Triangle and SI Joint Glide

Side Hip Glide and Shear

Upper Back Glide, Shear, and Rinse

Base of Skull Shear

Neck Decompress

Rest Reassess

Maps for Tennis, Golf, Boxing, Baseball/Softball, Lacrosse, Weightlifting/X-Games, Wrestling, Rock Climbing, Car Racing/Motocross, and Frisbee

All of these sports require excellent hand-eye coordination, stable footing, and grip control. Hip and knee stability is also required to move laterally and to manage upper body rotation.

Training Day Map (approximately 25 to 30 minutes)

Rest Assess

Performance Foot Treatment

Upper Body Rehydrate Sequence

Side Lying Arm Fans

Side Lying Backhand

> *Flip over and do Side Lying Arm Fans and Side Lying Backhand on the other side.*

Inner Thigh Lift

> *Flip over and do on the other side.*

SI Joint Shear

Hip to Heel Press

Figure 4

Pelvic Tuck and Tilt Challenge

Core Challenge

Rest Reassess

Game Day Map (approximately 12 minutes)

Rest Assess

Mini Performance Hand Treatment

Modified Tuck and Tilt Challenge

SI Joint Shear

Bent Knee Press

Hip to Heel Press

Rib Length *(to assess rib motion)*

Upper Back Glide and Shear

Arm Glide and Shear

Upper Back Rinse

Rib Length

Rest Reassess

Maps for Running, Biking, Track and Field, Surfing, Skateboarding, and Swimming

All of these sports require that you're nimble, quick on your feet, and have adequate rotation in your torso. These Maps will improve shoulder stability by restoring torso mobility, core control, and pelvic stability.

Training Day Map (approximately 25 minutes)

Rest Assess

Performance Foot Treatment

Rib Length *(to assess rib motion)*

Upper Back Glide and Shear

Inner Shoulder Blade Glide and Shear

Side Rib Glide and Outer Shoulder Blade Glide and Shear

Upper Back Rinse

Rib Length

Side Hip Glide and Shear

Side Leg Lift

SI Joint Shear

Pelvic Tuck and Tilt Challenge

Core Challenge

Mini Bridge

Figure 4

Low Back Decompress

Rest Reassess

Game Day Map (approximately 12 minutes)

Rest Assess

Mini Performance Foot Treatment

Seated Compression Sequence

Rib Length

Base of Skull Shear

Neck Decompress

Rest Reassess

▶ Pain and Joint Injury Maps

It goes without saying that athletics can lead to injury. I've devised three MELT Performance Maps for three categories that focus on specific joints to restore joint centralization and stability. If you don't currently have pain but want to reduce your risk of injury on your total rest and recovery days, try one of these MELT Maps to keep your body pain-free.

When it comes to dealing with pain, I recommend taking the Indirect Before Direct approach. Rather than focusing on the area of pain, MELT other parts of your body first. This indirectly rehydrates the troubled area without overstressing the nervous system. This is without a doubt the most effective way to eliminate pain.

Even though the Maps begin indirectly, they do directly treat the region of your body that has pain. If you find that doing the Map the first time or two increases your sensitivity, go more indirect by trying one of the other Maps below and then come back to the focused, direct Map again in a week. Giving your body more indirect treatments may take longer, but it will improve your results and make more lasting changes.

Map for Neck, Shoulders, and Elbows (approximately 25 minutes)

If you have suffered an injury, have had surgery, or have persistent pain in your upper body, this is a direct Map to address these three primary spaces of your upper body and restore stability to your shoulder girdle.

Rest Assess

Performance Hand Treatment

Upper Body Stability Sequence:

Rib Length *(to assess rib motion)*

Upper Back Glide and Shear

Inner Shoulder Blade Glide and Shear

Arm Glide and Shear

Side Lying Arm Fans

Side Lying Backhand

Rib Length *(to reassess rib motion)*

Neck Release Sequence

Base of Skull Shear

Neck Decompress

Rest Reassess

Map for Low Back, Hip Joints, and SI Joints (approximately 25 minutes)

If you have suffered an injury, have had surgery, or have persistent pain in your low back, pelvis, or hip joints, this is a direct Map to address pelvic stability and restore control to your NeuroCore.

Rest Assess

Performance Foot Treatment

Modified Tuck and Tilt Challenge

SI Joint Shear

Bent Knee Press

Pelvic Tuck and Tilt Challenge

Core Challenge

Low Back Decompress

Mini Bridge

Side Leg Lift

Rest Reassess

Map for Knee, Ankle, and Foot Pain (approximately 25 minutes)

If you have suffered an injury, have had surgery, or have shin splints or persistent pain, cramping, or swelling in your lower body, this is a direct Map to address timing and control and restore stability in your hip, knee, and ankle joints.

Rest Assess

Performance Foot Treatment

Seated Compression Sequence

Clams

Inner Thigh Lift

SI Joint Shear

Bent Knee Press

Figure 4

Hip to Heel Press

Rest Reassess

▶ Lifestyle Maps

Whether you spend most of your time in a seated position, you're on your feet all day, or your job requires heavy lifting, these MELT Maps will help keep your body stable and mobile and your joints free of pain.

The Desk Jockey (approximately 20 minutes)

If you're seated for more than two hours a day, this MELT Map will help reduce your "desk sentence." Seriously, we are sitting ourselves to death. The seated posture decreases the supportive qualities of fascia, reduces blood flow, and increases blood pressure and your chances of developing heart disease and diabetes. On top of doing this Map, try to get out of your chair at least every forty-five minutes for just a minute and reach both arms up over your head with a deep inhale and drop them to your sides as you exhale; do this four to five times. You might look a little silly at work, but your backside will thank you.

You can flip the two sequences around, or just do one to restore spinal stability and hip mobility. Remember to always start with a Rest Assess and end with a final Rest Reassess.

Option: Add a Mini Performance Hand Treatment to either sequence or do it on its own at work any time of the day.

Lower Body Sequence

Rest Assess

Tail Triangle and SI Joint Glide

SI Joint Shear

Bent Knee Press

Figure 4

Mini Bridge

Pelvic Tuck and Tilt Challenge

Core Challenge

Low Back Decompress

Rest Reassess

Upper Body Sequence

Rib Length *(to assess rib motion)*

Upper Back Glide and Shear

Upper Back Rinse

Side Lying Backhand

Rib Length *(to reassess rib motion)*

Base of Skull Shear

Neck Decompress

Rest Reassess

The Manual Laborer (approximately 20 minutes)

If you have any manual labor job—such as construction, plumbing, working in a factory, or farming—or you're in the military, a firefighter, or an emergency responder, your low back and neck pay the price for the heavy gear you have to carry and the repetitive movements you do every day. I designed this MELT Map with all of you in mind. I want to help you sustain good shoulder and hip strength while also decompressing your neck and low back. You can do both of these sequences back to back, or do one every other day for best results.

Option: Add any of the Performance Hand or Foot Treatments to one or both sequences depending on how much time you have for your self-care practice.

Upper Body Sequence

Rest Assess

Upper Back Glide and Shear

Inner Shoulder Blade Glide and Shear

Arm Glide and Shear

Upper Back Rinse

Side Lying Arm Fans

Base of Skull Shear

Neck Decompress

Rest Reassess

Lower Body Sequence

SI Joint Shear

Pelvic Tuck and Tilt Challenge

Core Challenge

Bent Knee Press

Figure 4

Mini Bridge

Inner Thigh Lift

Rest Reassess

The Service Worker (approximately 20 minutes)

Whether you spend your days standing still or are on your feet and always on the move, this MELT Map is a must! Restaurant workers, retail workers, showroom managers, and salespeople are on their feet all day long, causing unnecessary pressure on their low backs. This can lead to aching feet, constantly stiff hips, and an inflexible low back. You can do both of these sequences back to back, or do one every other day.

Lower Body Sequence

Rest Assess

Performance Foot Treatment

Deep Hip Glide and Shear

Clams

SI Joint Shear

Bent Knee Press

Mini Bridge

Hip to Heel Press

Rest Reassess

Upper Body Sequence

Rib Length Assess

Performance Hand Treatment

Upper Back Glide and Shear

Upper Back Rinse

Rib Length Reassess

Rest Reassess

Glossary

MELT Performance and MELT Method Terminology

MELT: A simple self-treatment method that helps prevent pain, heal injury, and erase the negative signs of aging and active living. Using small balls for the hands and feet and a soft roller for the body, the MELT Method directly enhances body awareness, rehydrates connective tissue, and quiets the nervous system.

MELT Performance: Utilizing the Four Rs of the MELT Method and the Two Rs of NeuroStrength, this self-care system focuses on improving the quality of fascia and sustaining optimal sensorimotor control through self-administered techniques.

NeuroStrength: The principles that govern human sensory and motor integration, its plasticity, and its development. Movement is guided by sensory feedback and sensory expectation, and our sensations are determined by how we move. NeuroStrength utilizes and enhances the autonomic sensorimotor control that is often degraded by repetitive movements of everyday living and aging.

General Terms

Autopilot: The parts of our body that protect, support, and stabilize us without our voluntary control or conscious awareness.

Body Sense: The built-in "internal awareness meter" that allows the Autopilot to sense the body's position without the use of common senses. It's like the body's built-in GPS system, and like the Autopilot, it is involuntary and functioning all the time. A simplified term for proprioception and interoception.

Living Body Model: A dynamic functional model composed of five key elements focused on the autonomic aspects of healthy living, allowing you to assess and take care of yourself in a manner that is applicable to human beings rather than anatomical models. Simply put, the Living Body Model expresses the involuntary aspects of neurofascial function.

Masses and spaces: A structural assessment tool that simplifies complex anatomical terms. Used as reference points in all of the MELT moves to identify proper body position and placement. Instead of having to think about a femur or hamstring, for instance, one just has to know that the head is a mass and the neck is a space. One of the rules of MELT is to only compress masses with the roller, we never compress the spaces.

NeuroCore: The mechanisms and reflexes that give us inherent stability without our conscious control. It's made up of the vast reflexes and neurological mechanisms that allow us to transfer load from the spine to the legs and move in an upright posture. The Reflexive Core stabilizes the spine and protects the organs, and the Rooted Core keeps the body grounded and mechanically helps sustain the primary masses (the head, ribs, and pelvis) over the feet.

Stuck stress: Dehydrated connective tissue or fascia that has lost its elasticity. Stuck stress accumulates from the normal repetition of the moves we make in our daily lives.

Tensional energy: The hydrostatic potential that exists in the connective tissue fluid matrix that creates head-to-toe tensional integrity and helps to keep the body's masses balanced over a small base of support (the feet). It is achieved through the MELT Rehydrate techniques of Rinsing and Lengthening, which move local fluid globally through the fascia and into the pre-lymphatic channels. This model simplifies scientific terms such as interstitial fluid flow, mechanotransduction, piezoelectricity, and tensegrity.

MELT Move Terms

Compression: A tolerable, gentle pressure used to stimulate fluid exchange between cells or within the extracellular matrix.

Decompress: To regain integrity and stability in joints or primary spaces such as the neck or low back by creating fluid exchange and then releasing the fluid into the joint spaces.

Differentiation: Moving one mass of the body in isolation while keeping surrounding masses stable. This is different from isolating movement with a focus on what's moving; differentiation is used to describe focusing on what's staying stable as one moves a single mass to reacquire proper motor control.

Extensibility: The ability of tissue to extend to a limited threshold to reduce the potential of tearing in both muscles and connective tissue. The ability to adapt to spatial length.

Focused breath: Focusing the breath toward the part of the body one is compressing, or inhaling with conscious thought. This stimulates receptors in the tissues and helps blood and fluid circulate throughout the body.

Four Rs: The direct and indirect techniques of MELT: Reconnect, Rebalance, Rehydrate, and Release. The Four Rs are the "recipe" for eliminating stuck stress, and the MELT protocol for self-treatment. Within each category, different techniques are used to achieve desired results.

Friction: A very light, random movement that stimulates the superficial connective tissues and encourages fluid movement in the connective tissue and lymphatic and capillary systems. Friction is done on the hands and feet only.

Gliding: A two-directional movement using consistent pressure where a ball or roller is moved under a small surface area of the body to prepare the tissue for the next move, called Shearing, and to investigate for tenderness and dehydration.

Map: MELT Maps combine a series of sequences to create a complete self-treatment protocol that includes the Four Rs of MELT and the Two Rs of NeuroStrength. Maps can include a mix of basic, intermediate, and advanced sequences, some using NeuroStrength for improved performance, some using Rehydrate for recovery and prevention.

Move: The most basic element of MELT. A move applies techniques from one of the Four Rs to an area of the body.

Multitasking: As you acquire a movement pattern and find stability, you will be focusing on your set up, and what's staying stable as you move. You must multitask and spend a lot of time focusing on and thinking about many things to reintegrate. Multitasking distracts the mind, which is a part of creating new neural pathways, improved neuromotor control, and heightened sensory awareness.

Position Point Pressing: Mobilizes the many joints of the hands and feet, rejuvenating them with essential fluid. Increases the ease of mobility in the hands and feet, and improves the neural connection between the extremities and every other system of the body.

Rebalance: Techniques that enhance the control and timing of the Reflexive Core and Rooted Core (NeuroCore) mechanisms for improved balance and stability. Rebalancing techniques also recalibrate (or rebalance) the neurological regulators of stress and repair.

Reconnect: Techniques used to assess the body's current state before any MELT sequence or MELT Map is done, as well as after to reassess and value the changes that self-care can create. Reconnect moves also help the Autopilot reacquire its connection to the center of gravity, which heightens stability and efficiency in the autonomic regulators of the nervous system.

Rehydrate: Techniques that restore the fluid state and supportive qualities of the connective tissue system, relieve stuck stress, and improve tensional energy. These techniques improve the environment of all the joints, muscles, organs, and bones; they also decrease inflammation in the joints and improve the fluid and nutrient absorption of every cell in the body. Compression and Lengthening techniques are used to restore the elastic properties of the fascial system.

Release: Techniques to decompress unnecessary tension and compression in the neck and low back, as well as the joints of the spine, hands, and feet. Release techniques help restore the balance between masses and spaces and improve the mobility of the neck and low back space.

Rinsing: A slow, consistent, one-directional motion that improves the fluid flow (mechanotransduction) of the connective tissue system as a whole. Like moving water in a tub, Rinsing induces a vortex-like motion in the fluids of the body.

Sequence: A structured progression of MELT moves from two or more of the Four Rs that yields a specific result. Sequences allow one to reinforce MELT's unique approach of Indirect Before Direct, working indirectly toward regions of pain rather than attacking them with direct intervention.

Shearing: A smaller, specific movement with a ball or roller to stimulate a fluid exchange in connective tissue. Shearing requires a frictional engagement between layers within the body to improve the sliding and gliding surfaces at the interfaces of fascial layers.

Two-directional length: Using muscle to gently pull connective tissue in two directions at once to gain space in joints and hydrate the surrounding tissue.

Scientific Terminology

Adhesions: Bands of scar-like tissue that form between two surfaces inside the body.

Afferent nerve: Neurons that receive information from the sensory organs (e.g., eye, skin) and transmit this input to the central nervous system. An afferent nerve is also called a sensory nerve.

Biotensegrity: A biological model to define how bones float in fascia without touching one another and how the prestressed tension caused by fascia allows our body to manage tension and compression throughout the entire system.

Cell signaling: The process by which a cell receives and acts on an external chemical or physical signal, such as a hormone, thereby stimulating a specific cellular response.

Center of gravity: A point from which the weight of a body or system may be considered to act. In physics, it is an imaginary point in a body of matter where the total weight of the body may be thought to be concentrated. The concept is sometimes useful in predicting the behavior of a moving body when it is acted on by gravity. For the purposes of MELT, your center of gravity is in the center of your pelvic basin.

Collagen: An abundant protein, of which there are fourteen types, that constitutes a major component of fascia, giving it strength and flexibility.

Efferent nerve: Neurons that send impulses from the central nervous system to your limbs and organs.

Extracellular matrix: Any material produced by cells and excreted to the extracellular space within the tissues. It takes the form of both ground substance and fibers and is composed chiefly of fibrous elements, proteins involved in cell adhesion, and glycosaminoglycans and other molecules. It serves as a scaffolding, holding tissues together, and its form and composition help determine tissue characteristics.

Fascia: The soft tissue component of the connective tissue system. It interpenetrates and surrounds muscles, bones, organs, nerves, blood vessels, and other structures. Fascia is an uninterrupted three-dimensional web throughout the body. It is responsible for maintaining structural integrity and providing support and protection, and acts as a shock absorber. Fascia can refer to sheaths, joint capsules, organ capsules, muscular septa, ligaments, retinacula, aponeuroses, tendons, myofascia, neurofascia, and other fibrous collagenous tissues.

Homeostasis: The property of cells, tissues, and organisms that allows for the maintenance and regulation of the stability and constancy needed for proper functioning.

Hyaluronan: A glycosaminoglycan that is part of the extracellular matrix of synovial fluid, vitreous humor, cartilage, blood vessels, skin, and the umbilical cord. Along with lubricin, it maintains viscosity of the extracellular matrix, allowing for necessary lubrication of certain tissues.

Hydrostatic pressure: Relating to the equilibrium of liquids and the pressure exerted by liquid at rest. The pressure you apply is transmitted throughout the liquid in all directions equally.

Hypermobility, or laxity: A greater-than-normal range of motion in a joint, which may occur naturally or may be a sign of joint instability.

Inflammation: Part of the complex biological response of body tissues to harmful stimuli, such as pathogens, damaged cells, or irritants, and is a protective response involving immune cells, blood vessels, and molecular mediators.

Interstitial fluid: The extracellular fluid that bathes the cells of most tissues but which is not within the confines of the blood or lymph vessels and is not a transcellular fluid. It is formed by filtration through the blood capillaries and is drained away as lymph. It is the extracellular fluid volume minus the lymph volume, the plasma volume, and the transcellular fluid volume.

Involuntary action-reaction: Occurs without conscious choice or decision-making. Involuntary actions are the opposite of voluntary actions, which occur by choice. Involuntary actions, such as the heartbeat, breathing, hiccups, digestion, coughing, and sneezing, may or may not occur with the awareness of the organism performing them.

Ligament: A band of fascia that connects bones or supports viscera (the body's internal organs).

Lymphatic system: Responsible for the production, transport, and filtration of lymph fluid throughout the body. In addition to its important circulatory functions, the lymphatic system also has important immunological functions. Aspects of the lymphatics are part of the interstitium. Lymphatics regulate immunity and drive interstitial flow from fascia to the pre-lymphatic vessels.

Mechanoreceptors: Sensory receptors that respond to mechanical pressure or deformation.

Motor nerves: Nerves that carry command information out of the central nervous system and toward muscles or glands (effectors) that will execute the commands.

Nervous system: The collection of nerves and nerve cells (neurons) that transmit signals to and from different parts of the body. The autonomic nervous system (ANS) is the part of the nervous system responsible for control of the bodily functions that are not consciously directed, such as breathing, the heartbeat, and digestive processes. The enteric nervous system (ENS) is a subdivision of the ANS that directly controls the gastrointestinal system. The ENS is capable of autonomous functions such as the coordination of reflexes. It's estimated that there are between four hundred million and six hundred million neurons in the gut, working independently of the brain. The system produces about 95 percent of the serotonin and 50 percent of the dopamine found in the body. The parasympathetic nervous system (PNS) is sometimes called the rest and digest system because it conserves energy as it slows heart rate, increases intestinal and gland activity, and relaxes sphincter muscles in the gastrointestinal tract. The sympathetic nervous system (SNS) is a part of the ANS that serves to accelerate heart rate, constrict blood vessels, and raise blood pressure as needed. Its primary process is to stimulate the body's fight-or-flight response; however, it is constantly active at a basic level to maintain homeostasis.

Neurofascial: Related to the inherent link between the autonomic nervous system and the fascial system.

Neuropathy: A functional disturbance or pathological change in the peripheral nervous system.

Neuroplasticity: How your brain is able to change as a result of experience.

Neurotransmitter: A chemical substance released at the end of a nerve fiber, causing the transfer of the impulse to another nerve fiber, a muscle fiber, or some other structure.

Nociception: The sensory nervous system's response to certain harmful or potentially harmful stimuli. A nociceptor is a sensory nerve cell that responds to damaging or potentially damaging stimuli by sending signals to the spinal cord and brain.

Pre-lymphatic channels: A conduit between the lymphatic system consisting of a network of thin-walled vessels that drains fluid and particular matter from the interstitial spaces to the lymphatic system. However, unlike blood vessels, the lymphatics do not form a circular system. The unidirectional lymph flow recovers fluid from the fascia and returns it to the cardiovascular system.

Proprioception: The sensory information that contributes to the sense of our position in space. It is often described as a sixth sense.

Proprioceptors (mechanoreceptors): The source of all proprioception. They detect any changes in physical displacement (movement or position) and any changes in tension, or force, within the body. They are found in all nerve endings of the joints, muscles, and tendons.

Tendon: A fibrous cord of fascia by which a muscle is attached to a bone.

Tensegrity: The property of materials made strong by the unison of tensioned and compressed parts. Tensional integrity, or floating compression, is a structural principle based on the use of isolated components in compression inside a net of continuous tension, in such a way that the compressed members do not touch each other and the prestressed tensioned members delineate the system spatially.

Recommended Reading

Research Papers and Abstracts

Alessandra C, Gonzalez A, Driscoll M, Schleip R, Wearing S, Jacobson E, Findley T, Klingler W. Frontiers in fascia research. *J Bodyw Mov Ther.* 2018; 22(4): 873–80.

Bordoni B, Zanier E. Skin, fascias, and scars: symptoms and systemic connections. *J Multidiscip Healthc.* 2014; 7: 11–24.

Cancelliero-Gaiad KM, Ike D, Pantoni CBF, Borghi-Silva A, Costa D. Respiratory pattern of diaphragmatic breathing and Pilates breathing in COPD subjects. *Braz J Phys Ther.* 2014; 18(4): 291–99. doi: 10.1590/bjpt-rbf.2014.0042.

Centers for Disease Control and Prevention. Nonfatal sports- and recreation-related injuries treated in emergency departments, United States, July 2000–June 2001. *MMWR Morb Mortal Wkly Rep.* 2002; 51: 736–40.

Chaudhry H, Schleip R, Ji Z, Bukiet B, Maney M, Findley T. Three-dimensional mathematical model for deformation of human fasciae in manual therapy. *J Am Osteopath Assoc.* 2008; 108(8):379–90.

Cowman MK, Schmidt TA, Raghavan P, Stecco A. Viscoelastic properties of hyaluronan in physiological conditions. *F1000Res.* 2015 Aug 25; 4: 622.

Critchley HD, Harrison NA. Visceral influences on brain and behavior. *Neuron.* 2013; 77(4): 624–38.

Fede C, Stecco C, Angelini A, Fan C, Belluzzi E, Pozzuoli A, Ruggieri P, De Caro R. Variations in contents of hyaluronan in the peritumoral micro-environment of human chondrosarcoma. *J Orthop Res.* 2019. doi: 10.1002/jor.24176.

Findley TW, Shalwala M. Fascia Research Congress: evidence from the 100 year perspective of Andrew Taylor Still. *J Bodyw Mov Ther.* 2013; 17(3): 356–64.

Friedl, P, Mayor R, Tuning Collective Cell Migration by Cell-Cell Junction Regulation, Cold Spring Harb Perspect Biol. 2017 Apr 3; 9(4). pii: a029199. doi: 10.1101/cshperspect.a029199. Review.

Gellhorn E. *Principles of Autonomic–Somatic Integration: Physiological Basis and Psychological and Clinical Implications.* Minneapolis: University of Minnesota Press, 1967.

Gordon CM, Andrasik F, Schleip R, Birbaumer N, Rea M. Myofascial triggerpoint release (MTR) for treating chronic shoulder pain: a new approach. *J Bodyw Mov Ther.* 2016; 00: 1–9.

Gordon CM, Birbaumer N, Andrasik F. Interdisciplinary fascia therapy (IFT method) reduces chronic low back pain: a pilot study for a new myofascial approach. Paper presented at the Ninth Interdisciplinary World Congress on Low Back and Pelvic Girdle Pain, Singapore, October 31–November 3, 2016.

Gordon CM, Graf C, Schweisthal M, Lindner SM, Birbaumer N, Montoya P, Andrasik F. Effects of self-help myofascial release tools: shearing versus rolling. CONNECT Congress: Connective Tissues in Sports Medicine, Congress Book 2017.

Gordon CM, Lindner SM, Birbaumer N, Montoya P, Andrasik F. Interdisciplinary fascia therapy (IFT) in chronic low back pain: an effectivity-outcome study with outpatients. Paper presented at Fascia Research IV, Washington, DC, November 2015, 253, and Ninth Interdisciplinary World Congress on Low Back and Pelvic Girdle Pain, Singapore, October 31–November 3, 2016.

Grimm D. Cell biology meets Rolfing. *Science.* 2007; 318: 1234–35. doi: 10.1126/science.318.5854.1234.

Grinnell F. Fibroblast mechanics in three-dimensional collagen matrices. *J Bodyw Mov Ther.* 2008; 12(3): 191–93. doi: 10.1016/j.jbmt.2008.03.005.

Haskell WL. Physical activity, sport, and health: toward the next century. *Res Q Exerc Sport* 1996; 67(suppl): 37–47.

Henley CE, Ivins D, Mills M, Wen FK, Benjamin BA. Osteopathic manipulative treatment and its relationship to autonomic nervous system activity as demonstrated by heart rate variability: a repeated measures study. *Osteopath Med Prim Care.* 2008; 2: 7. doi: 10.1186/1750-4732-2-7.

Ingber D. Tensegrity and mechanotransduction. First International Fascia Research Congress, Boston, 2007. DVD recording available from http://fasciacongress.org/2007/.

Ingber DE. From cellular mechanotransduction to biologically inspired engineering: 2009 Pritzker Award Lecture, BMES Annual Meeting October 10, 2009. *Ann Biomed Eng.* 2010; 38(3): 1148–61. doi: 10.1007/s10439-010-9946-0.

Johansson H, Sjölander P, Sojka P. Receptors in the knee joint ligaments and their role in the biomechanics of the joint. *Crit Rev Biomed Eng.* 1991; 18(5): 341–68.

Kruger L. Cutaneous sensory system. In: Adelman G. (ed.). *Encyclopedia of Neuroscience,* Vol. 1, 293–295. Boston: Birkhauser.

Langevin HM. Fibroblast cytoskeletal remodeling contributes to viscoelastic response of areolar connective tissue under uniaxial tension. Second International Fascia Research Congress, 2009. DVD recording available from: http://fasciacongress.org/2009/.

Lee DG. Treatment of pelvic instability. In: Vleeming A, Mooney V, Dorman T, Snijders C, Stoeckart R (eds.). *Movement, Stability and Low Back Pain,* 593–615. Edinburgh: Churchill Livingstone.

Lee DG, Vleeming A. Impaired load transfer through the pelvic girdle: a new model of altered neutral zone function. In: Proceedings from the Third Interdisciplinary World Congress on Low Back and Pelvic Pain, Vienna, Austria, 1998, 76–82.

Legrain V, Guérit JM, Bruyer R, Plaghki L. Attentional modulation of the nociceptive processing into the human brain: selective spatial attention, probability of stimulus occurrence, and target detection effects on laser evoked potentials. *Pain.* 2002; 99: 21–39.

Legrain V, Iannetti GD, Plaghki L, Mouraux A. The pain matrix reloaded: a salience detection system for the body. *Prog Neurobiol.* 2011; 93(1): 111–24.

Lewis JS, Kersten P, McCabe CS, McPherson KM, Blake DR. Body perception disturbance: a contribution to pain in complex regional pain syndrome (CRPS). *Pain.* 2007; 133: 111–19.

Marshall SW, Guskiewicz KM. Sports and recreational injury: the hidden cost of a healthy lifestyle. *Inj Prev.* 2003; 9: 100–102.

Melzack R. Pain and the neuromatrix in the brain. *J Dent Educ.* 2001; 65: 1378–82.

Moseley GL. Why do people with complex regional pain syndrome take longer to recognize their affected hand? *Neurology.* 2004; 62: 2182–86.

Moseley GL, Hodges PW. Loss of normal variability in postural adjustments is associated with non-resolution of postural control after experimental back pain. *Clin J Pain.* 2004; 21:323–329.

Reed RK, Liden A, Rubin K. Edema and fluid dynamics in connective tissue remodeling. *J Mol Cell Cardiol.* 2010; 48(3): 518–23. doi: 10.1016/j.yjmcc.2009.06.023.

Rutkowski JM, Swartz MA. A driving force for change: interstitial flow as a morphoregulator. *Trends Cell Biol.* 2007; 17(1): 44–50. doi: 10.1016/j.tcb.2006.11.007.

Sanjana F, Chaudhry H, Findley T. Effect of MELT method on thoracolumbar connective tissue: the full study. *J Bodyw Move Ther.* 2016; 21(1): 179–85. http://dx.doi.org/10.1016/j.jbmt.2016.05.010.

Schleip R. Fascial plasticity: a new neurobiological explanation, part 1 and 2. *J Bodyw Move Ther.* 2003; 7(1): 11–19.

Seminowiz DA, Mikulis DJ, Davis KD. Cognitive modulation of pain-related brain responses depends on behavioral strategy. *Pain.* 2004; 112: 48–58.

Snijders CJ, Vleeming A, Stoeckart R. Transfer of lumbosacral load to iliac bones and legs: Part 1: Biomechanics of self-bracing of the sacroiliac joints and its significance for treatment and exercise. *Clin Biomech.* 1993; 8(6): 285–94.

Stecco A, Gesi M, Stecco C, Stern R. Fascial components of the myofascial pain syndrome. *Curr Pain Headache Rep.* 2013 Aug; 17(8): 352.

Stecco A, Stern R, Fantoni I, De Caro R, Stecco C. Fascial disorders: Implications for treatment. *PM R.* 2016 Feb; 8(2): 161–68. doi: 10.1016/j.pmrj.2015.06.006.

Stecco C, Fede C, Macchi V, Porzionato A, Petrelli L, Biz C, Stern R, De Caro R. The fasciacytes: A new cell devoted to fascial gliding regulation. *Clin Anat.* 2018 Jul; 31(5): 667–76.

Theise N, et al. Structure and distribution of an unrecognized interstitium in human tissues, *Sci Rep.* 2018; 8(1): 4947. doi: 10.1038/s41598-018-23062-6.

US Department of Health and Human Services. *Physical Activity and Health: A Report of the Surgeon General.* Atlanta: US Department of Health and Human Services, Centers for Disease Control and Prevention, National Center for Chronic Disease Prevention and Health Promotion, 1996, 3–8, 142–44.

Vagedes J, Gordon CM, Mueller V, Andrasik F, Gevirtz R, Schleip R, Birbaumer N. Anxiety correlates with the reactive but not with the sensory dimension of the brief pain inventory within patients with chronic lower back pain: a prospective cross-sectional study. Paper presented at the Ninth Interdisciplinary World Congress on Low Back and Pelvic Girdle Pain, Singapore, October 31–November 3, 2016.

Vagedes J, Gordon CM, Mueller V, Andrasik F, Gevirtz R, Schleip R, Birbaumer N. Comparison of myofascial-trigger-point-release and core stabilization exercises on range of motion within patients with chronic low back pain: a randomized, controlled trial. Paper presented at the Ninth Interdisciplinary World Congress on Low Back and Pelvic Girdle Pain, Singapore, October 31–November 3, 2016.

Vagedes J, Gordon CM, Müller V, Beutinger D, Radtke M, Andrasik F, Gevirtz R, Schleip R, Hautzinger M, Birbaumer N (eds.). Myofascial-trigger-point-release and paced breathing training for chronic low back pain: a randomized controlled trial. In: *Fascia Research II: Basic Science and Implications for Conventional and Complementary Health Care.* Munich: Elsevier, 2009, 249.

Van der Wal J. The architecture of the connective tissue in the musculoskeletal system: an often overlooked functional parameter as to proprioception in the locomotor apparatus. *Int J Ther Massage Bodywork.* 2009; 2(4): 9–23.

Vetrugno R, Liguori R, Cortelli P, Montagna P. Sympathetic skin response: basic mechanisms and clinical applications. *Clin Auton Res.* 2003; 13(4): 256–70.

Vleeming A, Pool-Goudzwaard AL, Hammudoghlu D, Stoeckart R, Snijders CJ, Mens JM. The function of the long dorsal sacroiliac ligament: its implication for understanding low back pain. *Spine.* 1996; 21(5): 556–62.

Vleeming A, Pool-Goudzwaard AL, Stoeckart R, van Wingerden JP, Snijders CJ. The posterior layer of the thoracolumbar fascia: its function in load transfer from spine to legs. *Spine.* 1995; 20: 753–58.

Vleeming A, Volkers ACW, Snijders CJ, Stoeckart R. Relation between form and function in the sacroiliac joint. 2: Bio-mechanical aspects. *Spine.* 1990; 15(2): 133–36.

Ward RC. Integrated neuromusculoskeletal release and myofascial release. In: Ward RC (ed.). *Foundations for Osteopathic Medicine*, 2nd ed., 931–65. Philadelphia: Lippincott Williams & Wilkins, 2002.

Watkins LR, Maier SF, Goehler LE. Immune activation: the role of pro-inflammatory cytokines in inflammation, illness responses and pathological pain states. *Pain.* 1995; 63: 289–302.

Yahia L, Rhalmi S, Newman N, Isler M. Sensory innervation of human thoracolumbar fascia: an immunohistochemical study. *Acta Orthop Scand.* 1992; 63(2): 195–97.

Zullow M, Reisman S. Measurement of autonomic function during craniosacral manipulation using heart rate variability. In: Proceedings of the 1997 IEEE 23rd Northeast Bioengineering Conference, Durham, NH, May 21–22, 1997. New York: IEEE, 1997, 83–84.

Books and Articles

Avison, J. *Yoga: Fascia, Anatomy and Movement.* Edinburgh, UK: Handspring Publishing, 2015.

Butler, David, and Moseley, Lorimer. *Explain Pain.* 2nd ed. Adelaide, Australia: Noigroup, 2013.

Chaitow, L. *Soft Tissue Manipulation: A Practitioner's Guide to the Diagnosis and Treatment of Soft Tissue Dysfunction and Reflex Activity.* Rochester, VT: Healing Arts Press, 1988.

Cottingham, J. T. *Healing Through Touch: A History and a Review of the Physiological Evidence.* Boulder, CO: Rolf Institute Publications, 1985.

Dalton, E. *Advanced Myoskeletal Alignment Techniques for Shoulder, Arm, and Hand Pain*, Vol. 3. Tulsa, OK: Freedom from Pain Institute, 2006.

——. *Myoskeletal Alignment for Hip, Low Back, and Leg Pain.* Tulsa, OK: Freedom from Pain Institute, 2006.

Franklin, Eric N. *Dynamic Alignment Through Imagery.* 2nd ed. Champaign, IL: Human Kinetics, 2012.

Frederick, A. and C. Frederick. *Fascial Stretch Therapy.* Edinburgh, UK: Handspring Publishing, 2014.

Greenman, Philip E. *Principles of Manual Medicine.* 2nd ed. Baltimore: Lippincott Williams & Wilkins, 1996.

Guimberteau, Jean-Claude, and C. Armstrong. *Architecture of Human Living Fascia: Cells and Extracellular Matrix as Revealed by Endoscopy.* Pencaitland, Scotland: Handspring, 2015.

Hedley, Gil. "Reconsidering the Fuzz: Notes on Distinguishing Normal and Abnormal Fascial Adhesions." In: Dalton, Erik, and Judith Aston (eds.). *Dynamic Body: Exploring Form, Expanding Function*, 62–73. Free from Pain Institute, 2011.

Hitzmann, Sue. *The MELT Method: A Breakthrough Self-Treatment System to Eliminate Chronic Pain, Erase the Signs of Aging, and Feel Fantastic in Just 10 Minutes a Day!* New York: HarperOne, 2013.

Kapandji, I. A. *Physiology of the Joints.* New York: Churchill Livingstone, 1971.

Kendall, Florence Peterson, Elizabeth Kendall McCreary, Patricia Gelse Provance, Mary McIntyre Rodgers, and William Anthony Romani. *Muscles: Testing and Function with Posture and Pain.* 5th ed. Baltimore: Lippincott Williams & Wilkins, 2005.

Koch, Liz. *Core Awareness: Enhancing Yoga, Pilates, Exercise and Dance.* Berkeley, CA: North Atlantic Books, 2012.

——. *The Psoas Book.* 30th anniversary rev. ed. Felton, CA: Guinea Pig Publications, 2012.

——. *Stalking Wild Psoas: Embodying Your Core Intelligence.* Berkeley, CA: North Atlantic Books, 2019.

Larkam, Elizabeth. *Fascia In Motion: Fascia-Focused Movement for Pilates.* Edinburgh, UK: Handspring Publishing, 2017.

Miller, Jill. *The Roll Model*. Las Vegas, Nevada: Victory Belt Press, 2014.

Myers, Thomas W. *Anatomy Trains: Myofascial Meridians for Manual and Movement Therapists*. 3rd ed. New York: Churchill Livingstone, 2014.

Netter, F. H. *The Nervous System*. New York: Ciba Pharmaceuticals, 1953.

Pollack, Gerald H. *The Fourth Phase of Water: Beyond Solid, Liquid, and Vapor*. Seattle: Ebner and Sons, 2013.

——. *Muscles and Molecules: Uncovering the Principles of Biological Motion*. Seattle: Ebner and Sons, 1990.

Stecco, Carla. *Functional Atlas of the Human Fascial System*. London: Elsevier, 2015.

Websites

Dalton, Erik. "Core Myoskeletal Alignment Techniques for Head-to-Toe Treatment," https://erikdalton.com

Hedley, Gil. Integral Anatomy, https://www.gilhedley.com

Hitzmann, Sue. MELT Method, https://www.meltmethod.com

Journal of Bodywork and Manual Therapy, https://www.bodyworkmovement therapies.com

Lee, Diane. https://www.DianeLee.ca

Myers, Thomas. Anatomy Trains, https://www.anatomytrains.com

National Institutes of Health, https://www.nih.gov

PubMed, https://www.ncbi.nlm.nih.gov/pubmed

Research Gate, https://www.researchgate.net

Schierling, Russell. http://www.doctorschierling.com

Schleip, Robert. https://www.fasciaresearch.com

Acknowledgments

I was lucky enough to have Leon Chaitow as a teacher, adviser, and mentor. His teaching went so far beyond anything I'd learned during my master's program. His influence inspired me to take a more holistic view on everything from pain to movement and was my introduction into the world of osteopathic therapy. His contributions, including his writing and as Editor in Chief of the *Journal of Bodywork and Movement Therapies*, are that of a legend and icon. On September 20, 2018, Leon passed away surrounded by family. His loss is felt deeply.

His role at the *JBMT* has been passed down to Jerrilyn Cambron, and with his daughter Sasha Cohen as Managing Director, she will sustain his vision of the *JBMT* as a scientifically rigorous venue for interdisciplinary dialogue, lifelong professional development, and educational support for practitioners and students. His legacy lives on in his many books and articles, in the students he taught, in the patients he treated, and in the family to whom he was a devoted and beloved husband and father. The greatest way to honor him is to continue to carry that torch. I hope to do that each time I work with a client and with the techniques I share in this book. I am so grateful for his encouragement and belief in me.

A special thanks to Erik Dalton for taking on the task of writing the foreword to this book after Leon's passing. Beyond helping me refine my hands-on skills with his inspirational teaching, Erik is a pioneer and a brilliant educator, and much like Leon, is blessed with passion, kindness, and a sense of humor.

I want to express my deepest gratitude to my clients and students over the past thirty years of practice and teaching, most especially the original MELT Tribe at the JCC in Manhattan. The dedicated weekly practice and transformation I've witnessed with my own eyes year after year have been integral to the development of this method of self-care.

To my small but dedicated business team who work tirelessly to share the MELT message, I am forever grateful for your talent and tenacity. A special thanks to Karen Moline and Sara Bethell for shaping this book into a user-friendly manuscript that anyone can benefit from. Sara, your editing skills are that of a Jedi master. Special thanks to Jaci Dygos for taking on so much and sticking with me to complete "one more project." The leadership and talent you and the rest of our business team—Allison, Michelle, Monique, Magz, and Lewann—have brought to Longevity Fitness is astounding, and truly, I'm forever grateful to all of you for your belief in me.

I feel so blessed to be a part of the growing field of fascial research. This international community of like-minded "somanauts" (as Gil Hedley calls those who explore inner space) has shed light on the cellular world and importance of fascia as it relates to neurological function and overall healthy living. A special thanks to the Fascia Research Society, the Fascia Research Congress, and pioneers such as Thomas Findley, MD, PhD; Gil Hedley, PhD; Leon Chaitow, DO, ND; Erik Dalton, PhD; Robert Schleip, PhD; Jean Claude Guimberteau, MD; Carla Stecco, MD; and the vast number of neuroscientists, fascial researchers, and therapists who have brought so much rich science to the forefront of this community and have been so supportive in my pursuit of helping others live a more active, happy, and healthy life. To list all of them would fill pages. I feel privileged to share these insights in this and my previous book and thankful for all of the support over the years. I hope to be the "connective tissue" between these true scientific pioneers and the general public.

A special thanks to Brian Leighton for the many photo shoots (and reshoots) needed to help people visualize the specificities of each MELT move, and, of course, for your friendship and love over the years. Thank you to Phil Widlanski for giving me my studio to create and practice in, and for believing in me and making me a part of your family. And a special thanks to my friends and family for your belief in me.

Thank you to the hundreds of MELT instructors who have shared the MELT message and changed lives, including my own. Your curiosity and dedication are unwavering. I've learned so much from each and every one of you and am so proud of what you've all accomplished in sharing this method of self-care with so many beyond my physical reach.

Thank you to Gideon Weil, my editor at HarperOne, for the opportunity to create a second book and for seeing the potential of MELT Performance. His belief in me and my vision is extraordinary. Thanks to Lisa Zuniga and the HarperOne team for all of your hard work to help me bring this potential into reality. I'm so appreciative for the support and encouragement.

Thanks to all of you for being part of the MELT Tribe.

Index

dehydration: causing inhibition of stabilizers, 187; cell, 68. *See also* hydration

dementia, 27

depression, 27

dermatitis, 64

Desk Jockey Map, 295–96

diaphragm: cause of shoulder pain, 53; Rest Assess and Rest Reassess, 125; restoring motion through the Rebalance Sequence, 110; stuck stress in the, 127

differentiation, 159, 300

digestion: cycle of inflammation and, 64; description and process of the, 63; enteric nervous system or gut regulator of, 63–64; use NeuroStrength to help regulate your, 57–68

Direct Shearing technique, 115

disease: how stress makes one vulnerable to, 57; research findings on fascia relationship to, 100–101. *See also* health status

doctors: neuroplasticity not studies by, 43–44; practice cure using a symptom-based practice, 43

The Dr. Oz Show(TV show), 104–5

elbow pain, 6, 293

"emotional brain" (limbic system), 75

emotional distress: childhood fears bringing, 84, 88; how the past shapes your present, 79–85; post-9/11, 12, 71; of post-traumatic stress disorder (PTSD) and pain, 12, 77, 82; somato-emotional release, 77–79; why physical pain can be caused by, 74–79. *See also* trauma

emotional foundation: building a, 87–89; strengthening your emotional resilience, 89–92; unconditional love and support power for, 88–89

emotional posturing, 76

emotional resilience: change your mind to change your body, 91–92; description of, 89; NeuroStrength for reconnecting and tuning in to our, 90–91; sources of, 89–90

emotional state: how our history and perceptions impact our, 71–74; pain as both a sensory and an, 52–55; region of brain responsible for both movement and, 75–79

energy: how fascia stores, 26; Tensional Energy, 98–99

enteric nervous system (ENS), 61, 63–65, 303

epilepsy, 27

exercise: does not necessarily improve stability, 3–4; preconceived notion the injuries are "fixed" by, 50; understanding how it affects the body, 57. *See also* active lifestyle

extensibility, 300

extension, 39

extracellular matrix (ECM), 24–25, 100, 302

fasciacytes, 100

fascia/fascial system: biomechanics and immune system support by, 100–101; definition of, 24, 302; energy stored by, 26; as the internal environment, 23–26, 79–80, 102; fasciacytes cells of, 100; how it leverages and disperses force laterally, 191–92; how MELT's soft roller and balls help to rehydrate, 102; how neurological stability is linked to, 25–26; how sitting affects your, 50–51; how we store memory in the, 76–77; hydration required for healthy, 26; link between autonomic function and dysfunction, 101–2; resilient, 102; superficial, 55–56. *See also* connective tissue

fascial bias, 5

somato-emotional release, 77–79

spiderweb/cobweb analogy, 50

spinal mobility: NeuroCore Stability Sequence goal of improving, 245; NeuroCore Stability Sequence moves for, 246–55

Sports Performance Maps, 287, 288–93

stability: connective tissue (or fascial system) providing the body with, 4–5; how repetitive movements cause injuries interfering with, 1–3; learned during infancy, 37; MELT Performance providing needed, 2–3, 9–10, 20–21; NeuroCore for whole-body, 106–7; NeuroCore Stability Sequence to improve, 113, 245–55; Reintegrate and Repattern to restore, 183–85; strength of muscles as only one factor in, 3–4; training to improve, 1; understanding the science of, 28–29. See also motor control systems; NeuroStrength (neurological stability)

stability maps: Lifestyle Maps, 287, 295–98; Pain and Joint Injury Maps, 287, 293–95; Sports Performance Maps, 287, 288–93. See also MELT Maps

stabilizing mechanisms: conditions that inhibit, 187–88; how the Two Rs prevent inhibition of, 188–98; involuntary, slow-twitch vs. voluntary, fast-twitch muscle fibers, 185, 187; pelvic and shoulder, 185, 186, 187

Stecco, Carla, 100

Still, Andrew Taylor, 5

strength training, 3–4

stress: "fight, flight, or freeze" response to, 86; impact on general health by, 57; PTSD (post-traumatic stress disorder), 12, 77, 82, 87; use NeuroStrength to regulate your levels of, 57–68. See also stuck stress

structural strength: description and joint stability function of, 28, 30–31; difference between muscle strength and, 30–31

stuck stress: association between pain and, 53; definition of, 299; description and causes of, 5, 20; as the heart of the MELT Method, 183; how repetition creates, 47; how to identify in your own body, 127; neurological stability and control systems effected by, 5, 29; Reconnect techniques to assess and address, 103–6. See also stress

sudden chronic pain, 12, 54

superficial fascia, 55–56

surfing, 292

swimming, 292

sympathetic nervous system (SNS), 62–63, 65–66

Tail Triangle and SI Joint Glide, 123, 173, 276

tennis, 3, 12, 40, 45, 135, 186, 288, 290

tensegrity, 31, 303

Tensional Energy, 98–99, 300

Thiese, Neil, 101

thought virus: description of, 32; how it impacts neural networks of the brain, 82–84; undoing the power of the, 80–82

3-D Breath, 87, 108–11, 122

Tilt, Stack, and Roll, 215

Toe Lift Assess, 137

Toe Lift Reassess, 143–44

tonic muscles, 35–36

tonsillitis, 64

track and field, 292

Training Day Maps: description of, 287; for specific sports, 288–91, 292

trauma: hyperarousal and numbness responses to, 85–86; MELT Rebalance Sequence/3-D Breath Breakdown to deal with, 87; of 9/11, 12, 71; PTSD (post-traumatic stress disorder) response to, 12, 77, 82, 87; shame and helplessness